THE NEUROLOGY SHORT CASE

Second edition

Professor John GL Morris, DM (Oxon) FRCP FRACP

Chairman of the Education and Training
Committee of the Australian Association
of Neurologists

Past Examiner for the Royal Australasian College
of Physicians

Head of the Neurology Department,
Westmead Hospital, Sydney, NSW 2145, Australia

Clinical Professor, University of Sydney

Hodder Arnold

A MEMBER OF THE HODDER HEADLINE GROUP

First published in 1992 by Arnold
This second edition published in 2005, by Hodder Education,
a member of the Hodder Headline Group,
338 Euston Road, London NW1 3BH

http://www.hoddereducation.co.uk

Distributed in the United States of America by
Oxford University Press Inc.,
198 Madison Avenue, New York, NY10016
Oxford is a registered trademark of Oxford University Press

Whilst the advice and information in this book are believed to be true and
accurate at the date of going to press, neither the author[s] nor the publisher
can accept any legal responsibility or liability for any errors or omissions
that may be made. In particular (but without limiting the generality of the
preceding disclaimer), every effort has been made to check drug dosages;
however it is still possible that errors have been missed. Furthermore,
dosage schedules are constantly being revised and new side-effects
recognized. For these reasons the reader is strongly urged to consult the
drug companies' printed instructions before administering any of the drugs
recommended in this book.

British Library Cataloguing in Publication Data
A catalogue record for this book is available from the British Library

Library of Congress Cataloging-in-Publication Data
A catalog record for this book is available from the Library of Congress

ISBN-10:   0 340 88516 5
ISBN-13:   978 0 340 88516 1

1 2 3 4 5 6 7 8 9 10

Commissioning Editor: Joanna Koster
Development Editor: Sarah Burrows
Project Editor: Heather Fyfe
Production Controller: Lindsay Smith
Cover Design: Sarah Rees

Typeset in 11/15pt Adobe Minion by Servis Filmsetting Ltd, Manchester

Printed and bound in Malta

What do you think about this book? Or any other Hodder Arnold title?
Please visit our website at www.hoddereducation.co.uk

Contents

Foreword to the Second Edition

Professor Morris brings to life the art of clinical observation and examination in Neurology in this second edition of The Neurology Short Case. His clinical experience shines through in masterful discussions of common clinical scenarios supplemented with a rich array of video and still illustrations. This volume provides an essential companion when preparing for the MRCP or FRACP part 1 examinations. An experienced past examiner, Professor Morris, guides the reader through the common neurological problems encountered in short cases. His logical and clear approach, accompanied by sound advice, will be invaluable to candidates. In an era when the relevance of the clinical examination is under threat from technological advances, and the value of clinical signs is questioned in many areas of medicine, the importance of eliciting and interpreting clinical neurological signs remains unchallenged. The Neurology Short Case will therefore be of interest to the senior undergraduate and neurologist in training as a guide to the clinical neurological examination. Indeed, the consultant neurologist also will thoroughly enjoy Professor Morris's elegant descriptions of the art of examination, the many clinical pearls, and will more than likely find some new gems contained within this book.

Professor Philip Thompson
University Department of Medicine and Department of Neurology
University of Adelaide and Royal Adelaide Hospital

Foreword to the First Edition

If medical professional life were the Grand National the MRCP (or FRACP) would be Beecher's Brook – a daunting obstacle approached with caution, attempted with panic and surmounted with relief. Anything which makes this barrier less formidable, even to those on their third or fourth circuit of the course, is to be welcomed.

Dr Morris is a master of the old-fashioned art of clinical observation and examination and is renowned as a teacher of the subject. His wide experience both as practicing clinician, instructor and examiner, makes him a particularly suitable choice as an author of a book of this kind.

It is clearly written, well illustrated and full of sensible, practical guidance, not only to those taking examinations, for whom the neurology case is a particular dread, but for general physicians faced with everyday clinical problems. Even professional neurologists could scan its pages with profit and enjoyment.

Dr RW Ross Russell
Past President of the Association of British Neurologists

Preface to the Second Edition

This book is about the art of clinical examination in Neurology, the skills which neurologists use in everyday practice to assess their patients. Since it was first published in 1992, it has mainly found favour in candidates preparing for the FRACP clinical examination. It was also aimed at candidates preparing for the short case in the MRCP examination in the UK. The latter examination has now been replaced by PACES (Practical Assessment of Clinical Examination Skills) where the candidate is asked to assess a particular part of the nervous system, for example motor function in the legs, rather than deal with a specific symptom. The approach taken in this book, whereby the aspects of the examination which are most likely to be helpful in determining the site of the lesion and underlying cause, remains equally relevant to both forms of short case assessment.

In this new edition, the text has been revised to take account of helpful advice and criticism of the first edition, and many of the cases are now illustrated on video in the accompanying CD. New chapters have been included on involuntary movement disorders and assessing higher function. Some management issues are also listed in point form.

While the main target of this book remains candidates preparing for the FRACP and MRCP examinations, it may also prove useful for medical students and general practitioners wishing to hone their skills in the neurological examination.

John Morris, 2004

Preface to the First Edition

Most people studying for clinical vivas in medicine dread the neurology case. Unlike cardiology, respiratory medicine or gastroenterology there is no standard approach in neurology which is appropriate for most cases. In its entirety, the neurological examination is very time consuming; the skill lies in knowing which aspects of the examination deserve particular attention in a given case. This little book offers a simple approach to the assessment of a number of neurological problems which crop up in examinations and everyday practice.

Acknowledgements

I thank my colleagues for reading through the manuscript, sharing their clinical tips and giving suggestions and advice: Dr Elizabeth McCusker, Dr John King, Professor Christian Lueck, Dr Rick Boyle, Dr Mariese Hely, Dr Susie Tomlinson, Professor Philip Thompson, Dr Nicholas Cordato and Dr Victor Fung (who also helped greatly with the video material).

I am most grateful to Shanthi Graham (funded in part by the Westmead Charitable Trust), who has worked with me over many years on the video database and produced the video clips.

I also warmly acknowledge Dr Roly Bigg who, through his Movement Disorder Foundation, has provided financial support and encouragement to build the Video Database.

I would like to thank Faith Oxley for the figures which she drew and the following colleagues for their comments and advice on the first edition: Dr Leo Davies, Dr Jonathon Ell, Dr Ron Joffe, Dr Michael Katekar, Dr Jonathon Leicester, Dr Ivan Lorentz, Professor James McLeod, Dr Dudley O'Sullivan, Dr Ralph Ross Russell, Dr Tom Robertson, Dr Raymond Schwartz, Dr Ernest Somerville and Dr Grant Walker.

Abbreviations

ADM	abductor digiti minimi
ANA	antinuclear antibody
ANCA	anti-neutrophil cytoplasmic autoantibodies
ANF	anti-nuclear factor
APB	abductor pollicis brevis
A-R	Argyll Robertson
ASOT	anti-strepsolysin-O-antibody
AVM	arteriovenous malformation
COMT	catechol-ortho-methyltransferase
CPAP	continuous positive airway pressure
CPK	creatine phosphokinase
CRP	C-reactive protein
CSF	cerebrospinal fluid
CT	computed tomography
DCI	decarboxylase inhibitor
DI	dorsal interosseous
DLBD	diffuse Lewy body disease
DVT	deep vein thrombosis
ECG	electrocardiograph
EEG	electroencephalography
EMG	electromyography
ENA	extractable nuclear antigens
ESR	erythrocyte sedimentation rate
FBP	full blood picture
HIV	human immunodeficiency virus
INO	internuclear ophthalmoplegia
LFTs	liver function tests
MND	motor neurone disease
MRA	magnetic resonance angiography
MRI	magnetic resonance imaging

MSA	multiple system atrophy
PEG	percutaneous endoscopic gastrostomy
PSP	progressive supranuclear gaze palsy
SCA	spinocerebellar ataxia
SLE	systemic lupus erythematosus
SPECT	single-photon emission computed tomography
SSEPs	somatosensory evoked potentials
SSPE	subacute sclerosing panencephalitis
SSRIs	selective serotonin re-uptake inhibitors
VDRL	Venereal Disease Research Laboratories (test)

Picture Credits

Fig. 1.5   Adapted with permission from Fig. 27 of Aids to the Examination of the Peripheral Nervous System, London, Bailliere Tindall, 1986.

Fig. 1.6   Adapted with permission from Fig. 4.78a of Spillane J D and Spillane J A, An Atlas of Clinical Neurology, 3rd edn, Oxford, OUP, 1982.

Fig. 1.7   Adapted with permission from Fig. 76 of Aids to the Examination of the Peripheral Nervous System, London, Bailliere Tindall, 1986.

Fig. 1.8   Adapted with permission from Fig. 36 of Aids to the Examination of the Peripheral Nervous System, London, Bailliere Tindall, 1986.

Fig. 1.10 Adapted with permission from Fig. 87 of Aids to the Examination of the Peripheral Nervous System, London, Bailliere Tindall, 1986.

Fig. 2.1   Adapted with permission from Fig. 15 of Aids to the Examination of the Peripheral Nervous System, London, Bailliere Tindall, 1986.

Fig. 2.3   Adapted with permission from Fig. 72 of Aids to the Examination of the Peripheral Nervous System, London, Bailliere Tindall, 1986.

Fig. 3.1   Adapted with permission from Fig. 11 of Jamieson E B, Illustration of Regional Anatomy, Section VI, Edinburgh, E & S Livingston.

Fig. 3.2   Adapted with permission from Fig. 1 of Jamieson E B, Illustration of Regional Anatomy, Section VI, Edinburgh, E & S Livingston.

Fig. 4.1   Adapted with permission from Fig. 46 of Aids to the Examination of the Peripheral Nervous System, London, Bailliere Tindall, 1986.

Fig. 5.1   Adapted with permission from Fig. 4.34d of Spillane J D and Spillane J A, An Atlas of Clinical Neurology, 3rd edn, Oxford, OUP, 1982.

Fig. 5.2   Adapted with permission from Fig. 47 of Aids to the Examination of the Peripheral Nervous System, London, Bailliere Tindall, 1986.

Fig. 5.3   Adapted with permission from Fig. 83 of Aids to the Examination of the Peripheral Nervous System, London, Bailliere Tindall, 1986.

Fig. 5.4   Adapted with permission from Fig. 84 of Aids to the Examination of the Peripheral Nervous System, London, Bailliere Tindall, 1986.

Fig. 5.5   Adapted with permission from Fig. 2.11 of Donaldson J O, Neurology of Pregnancy, 2nd edn, W B Saunders, 1989.

Fig. 5.6   Adapted with permission from Fig. 89 of Aids to the Examination of the Peripheral Nervous System, London, Bailliere Tindall, 1986.

Fig. 5.7   Adapted with permission from Fig. 90 of Aids to the Examination of the Peripheral Nervous System, London, Bailliere Tindall, 1986.

Fig. 6.1   Adapted with permission from figures in Inman V., Human Locomotion, Canadian Medical Association Journal, 1966, 94, 1047—54.

Fig. 6.3   Both adapted with permission from Fig. 18.2 of Mumenthaler M, Neurological Differential Diagnosis, New York, Thierre-Stratton, 1985.

Fig. 7.1   Adapted with permission from Fig. 7.69 in Williams, P L, Warwick R, Functional Neuroanatomy of Man, Edinburgh, Churchill Livingston, 1986.

Fig. 9.1   Adapted with permission from Fig. 8.3 of McLeod J, Munro J (eds), Clinical Examination, 7th edn, Edinburgh, Churchill Livingston, 1986.

Fig. 9.3   Adapted with permission from Fig. 3.9 of Duus, P, Topical Diagnosis in Neurology, 2nd rvd edn, Stuttgart, Georg Thierne Verlay, 1983.

Fig. 12.1   Adapted with permission from Goodglass H, Kaplan, E, The Boston Diagnostic Aphasia Examination Booklet, Lea and Febinger, 1983.

"To study . . . disease without books is to sail an uncharted sea, while to study books without patients is not to go to sea at all".

William Osler

Introduction

As with any clinical examination, the neurology short case is a game with certain rules. You must understand these rules if you are to succeed. The aim of the game is to demonstrate your clinical skills in making a diagnosis in a limited amount of time. This demonstration will be much more impressive if you have a clear plan of action. Some candidates can evolve such a plan during the examination, but most need to have formulated a plan before-hand, usually in practice sessions. Before considering specific problems, a few general points are worth making.

Consideration for the patient

In the heat of the moment, it is easy to lose sight of the fact that you are dealing with a person as well as an interesting collection of signs. One of the reasons why clinical examinations retain their importance is that they provide an opportunity to see how you handle patients under difficult circumstances. Make a point of:

- Introducing yourself by name.
- Explaining to the patient what you are doing and what you want them to do, as you go along.
- Warning the patient before doing anything which might cause discomfort: eliciting the plantar or gag reflexes, using a pin to test pain sensation. A grunt of pain or a complaint by the patient will not impress the examiners.
- Putting the patient at their ease and taking every step to preserve their modesty and dignity.

The examiner's introduction

Take particular note of the introduction which the examiner gives. Considerable thought has often been given to this, and it is phrased in such a way as to direct you to the parts of the neurological examination which are most likely to be fruitful. With the introduction 'This patient has difficulty walking', for example, spend some time testing gait. Too often, with such a prompt, the candidate will allow the patient a couple of steps, and these viewed from close quarters, before embarking on a full examination on the couch.

The examiner expects you to go about your task in a systematic and thorough way. This introduces a conflict, for you only have 10 minutes or so in which to do it. A rushed examination is likely to lead to missed signs. A useful approach involves a careful and systematic examination of that part of the nervous system alluded to in the introduction, followed by simple screening tests of the remainder of the system (see below).

Technique

Neurological cases are favoured for clinical examinations because the signs, if correctly elicited, are obvious to examiner and candidate alike. The cases which are selected usually have good clinical signs. If a particular sign is subtle or doubtful it is better not to comment on it. In general, finding a sign which is not there is a greater sin than missing a sign which is there. The approach to examining the short case is important:

- **Inspection.** Always take time at the beginning of the examination to observe the patient as a whole. Note the skin, posture, facial expression, voice and any obvious clues such as muscle wasting, scars, bandages, drips or bladder drainage bags. If involuntary movements are present, note their distribution and whether they are regular in timing (tremor), rapid and irregular (chorea, tics, myoclonus, fasciculations) or slow and irregular (dystonia).
- **Tone** refers to the resistance encountered in muscles when the limbs are put through a range of **passive** movements. Unfortunately, many patients

try to make the doctor's task easier by actively moving their limbs during testing. Other patients resist the movements, particularly if they have not been put at ease. In the upper limbs, distract the patient by getting them repeatedly to extend and flex one arm at the shoulder while the other is being tested. A slight increase in tone occurs with this manoeuvre in normal subjects; in Parkinson's disease the increase is striking. A useful technique in the lower limb is, with the patient lying, to roll the leg at the hip and, occasionally and without warning, to lift the knee off the bed. If the heel also lifts off the bed, tone is increased. Describe the tone as normal or increased. Hypotonia is probably not a valid term, for in a fully relaxed normal subject no resistance is detectable to passive movement.

- **Muscle power** is tested using the techniques illustrated in *Aids to the Examination of the Peripheral Nervous System* (4th edition, WB Saunders, 2000). These are designed in such a way that, in most cases, you will overcome a particular muscle only if it is weak. This makes the assessment of muscle power more objective. Some muscles are more useful to test than others. It is good to get into the habit of testing muscles in a certain order as this will lessen the risk of leaving an important one out. The most useful muscles to test in the limbs are:

  - *Arms*: deltoid, biceps, triceps, brachioradialis, wrist extensors, finger extensors and flexors, abductor pollicis brevis, abductor digiti minimi and first dorsal interosseous.
  - *Legs*: gluteus maximus, iliopsoas, quadriceps, hamstrings, anterior tibial group, gastrocnemius/soleus, tibialis posterior and the peroneal muscles.

- **Coordination.** In the upper limbs, the most sensitive way of demonstrating *cerebellar incoordination* is to get the patient to try to slap their thigh alternately with the palm and back of the hand. The finger nose test is also useful. *Akinesia* due to Parkinson's disease is best tested by asking the patient to make piano-playing movements with the index and middle finger, or making a 'duck-bill' movement by repeatedly extending and flexing the fingers at the metacarpophalangeal joints. Lower-limb coordination is tested by getting the patient to walk and, on the couch, to run the heel up and down the shin.

  - Be careful how you discuss incoordination in a patient in whom you have demonstrated muscle weakness. Patients with weak muscles find tests of coordination difficult to perform. For the purposes of the short case examination, it is better to assume that incoordination, in the presence of muscle weakness, is due to that cause unless the weakness is minimal and the incoordination gross. Loss of proprioception may also cause incoordination.

- **Reflexes** are crucial to the formulation of a diagnosis, and their absence always requires an explanation. It is often difficult to elicit the ankle jerks in the elderly due to poor relaxation. Do not accept that a reflex is absent until you have done the Jendrassik reinforcement manoeuvre, or have tapped the Achilles tendon with the patient kneeling on a chair. For the upper-limb reflexes, get the patient to make a fist with the other hand, or clench the teeth; for the lower-limb reflexes, ask the patient to hook their hands together in a monkey grip and to try to pull them apart on command. The manoeuvre is most effective if the tendon is tapped immediately after the command to pull.

- **Sensory testing** is the least reliable aspect of the examination. Minor differences in sensation between different parts of the body are common, and are usually of no significance. Perception of sensation is also affected by whether the part of the body being tested is painful or weak. Many patients with, for example, Bell's palsy or trigeminal neuralgia (disorders not usually associated with sensory loss), will say that the skin on the affected side feels different.

  - More weight is given to a sensory disturbance if perception of a particular modality appears to be lost rather than altered. Ask the patient to say 'yes' each time the skin is lightly touched (with the eyes shut) and to distinguish between the blunt and sharp ends of a disposable pin applied repeatedly to an area of skin. In testing vibration, confirm that the patient really can feel the sensation by asking them when it stops. After a suitable pause, terminate the vibration by touching the end of the tuning fork.

  - For most neurological short cases, it is probably wise not to spend too much time on sensory testing early in the course of the examination. You have an opportunity, if time is running short, to tell the examiner that you would, under normal circumstances, now embark on a full examination of the sensory system and explain how this would be helpful.

- There are, however, circumstances in which you must make time to assess sensation:

  - A good starting point is to ask the patient if they have noticed any areas of numbness or tingling and to outline them.
  - In a patient with absent ankle jerks and an indwelling bladder catheter (suggesting a lesion of the cauda equina), it is essential to test sensation in the lower limbs and particularly in the buttocks.
  - In a patient with a spastic paraparesis, look for a sensory level. In testing pain perception use a disposable pin which, in the age of AIDS and viral hepatitis, you make a point of discarding at the end of the examination. If there is impaired sensation in the legs, establish the level at which this occurs, moving the stimulus repeatedly from the numb to the normal area. Test the front and back of the limbs and trunk. It is often useful to move a vibrating tuning fork (128 Hz) one segment at a time up the vertebral spines, or to drag the base up the legs and trunk and determine where it begins to feel cold. Cause the tuning fork to vibrate by plucking it between thumb and index. Banging it on the bed causes audible vibration and invalidates the test.
  - In a patient with suspected motor neurone disease, it is essential to show that sensation is normal.

- **Screening tests.** These are carried out in a few moments, and allow you to narrow down on a particular part or system for more detailed examination:

- *Face.* Make a point of observing the patient's facial expressions when you are being introduced. Listen to their voice. Look particularly for facial asymmetry, craniotomy scars, ptosis, baldness, squint or loss of expression.

- *Arms.* Ask the patient to put their arms out in front of them in the supine position, to hold their arms there for a few moments with the eyes shut, and then to touch their nose with each index finger in turn. This simple manoeuvre will often reveal important clues such as weakness, sensory loss, intention tremor, postural tremor, wrist drop and dystonia.

- *Legs.* Get the patient to walk in an open space. Observe the posture, arm swing and stride. Note whether the patient walks on a wide base or whether there is unsteadiness on turning. Ask the patient to walk heel to

toe. In a younger patient you may ask them to rise from a squatting position (testing proximal power) and to stand on their toes and heels
(testing distal power). Depending on what you find, you may also want to
test balance:

- *Romberg's sign* (see below).
- *The pull test* (see below).

- **Formulation of a diagnosis.** While you are examining the patient, you
  have two questions in mind: '*Where is the lesion*' and '*What is the likely
  underlying cause?*' In a short case you have little history, and your examination will therefore be mainly directed towards determining the site of
  the lesion. It should be clear to the examiner, from the aspects of the
  examination on which you concentrate, that these questions are being
  considered. You are not required to give a long list of likely causes. Indeed,
  the longer the list, the less well you have probably defined the problem.
  Nor are you expected to discuss the disease or its management in any
  detail. These are better tested by other means. Certain patterns of signs are
  useful in determining the site of the lesion:

- Generalized distal weakness is likely to be due to a peripheral neuropathy.
  Generalized proximal weakness is likely to be due to a myopathy.
- If a muscle is weak due to a peripheral nerve lesion, then all muscles
  innervated by that nerve below the site of the lesion will also be weak. For
  example, if brachioradialis is weak due to a lesion of the radial nerve in
  the spiral groove of the humerus, then extension of the fingers and wrist
  must also be weak. If they are not, then the problem must be elsewhere.
- In the case of an upper motor neurone disorder of the leg, the lesion must
  be above the level of the second lumbar vertebra. Whether the lesion is in
  the cord or above is determined by examining the upper limbs and
  cranial nerves. In the limited time available you may need to use your
  'screening' tests to determine this.
- If you have decided that the signs suggest a lower motor neurone disorder, it is helpful to consider whether the lesion is likely to be in the anterior horn cell, root, plexus, peripheral nerve, neuromuscular junction or
  muscle.
- In a cord lesion, reflexes are lost at the level of the lesion and increased
  below the lesion.

- In a unilateral brainstem lesion above the medulla, there may be 'crossed' signs with a cranial nerve lesion ipsilateral to the lesion and hemiparesis contralateral to the lesion.
- If the introduction and preliminary examination point to a lesion of the cerebral hemispheres (e.g. aphasia, sensory neglect or homonymous hemianopia), use your screening tests to see if there is a hemiparesis on the appropriate side.

Accepting that the neurology short case is a game, it must also be said that a sound approach to this game will do you no harm in dealing with patients in your clinical practice.

The wasted hand

1

Inspection
Distribution of wasting
Power, coordination and reflexes

Likely introduction: 'Weakness of the hand' or 'Examine the upper limb'.

The small muscles of the hand are supplied by the median and ulnar nerves and the C8/T1 roots. In a root lesion, all the small muscles are affected; in a single peripheral nerve lesion, wasting is selective.

Inspection

Upon noting wasting of the small muscles of the hand, check:

- **The patient's age.** Some loss of muscle bulk is normal in the elderly, but this is symmetrical in the two hands and the wasted muscles are not weak.
- **Arthritis.** This also causes wasting with minimal weakness (allowing for the pain which testing power may induce). Subluxation of the metacarpal bone of the thumb causes selective wasting of the thenar eminence which may be mistaken for a median nerve lesion.
- **Pupils.** A smaller pupil with ptosis (Horner's syndrome)[1] on the affected side suggests a C8/T1 root or cord lesion. Inequality of the pupils due to Horner's syndrome is most obvious in a dimly lit room.
- **Clawing** of the ring and little fingers (due to weakness of the lumbrical muscles) suggests an ulnar nerve lesion.
- **Fasciculations** suggest motor neurone disease.
- **Length of the two hands** and the size of the thumb nails. Hemi-atrophy (more accurately, hemi-smallness, as it reflects failure of growth rather

1. *Johann Friedrich Horner, Swiss ophthalmologist (1831–1886).*

than wasting) suggests injury to the nervous system in infancy (polio, birth trauma, stroke).

- **Scars** in the arms, especially over the elbow (ulnar nerve trauma).

Distribution of wasting

Take particular note of three muscles: abductor digiti minimi (ADM); first dorsal interosseous (1st DI); and abductor pollicis brevis (APB) (see Figs 1.1 and 1.2). There are three common patterns of wasting:

- *Wasting confined to APB.* Usually a median nerve lesion. Rarely due to cervical rib.
- *Wasting confined to ADM and 1st DI.* The patient has an ulnar nerve lesion.
- *Wasting of all three muscles.* Several possibilities (see below).

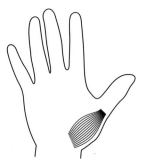

Figure 1.1 Abductor pollicis brevis.

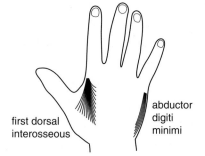

Figure 1.2 First dorsal interosseous and abductor digiti minimi.

Power, coordination and reflexes

After the arm raising screening test, test power in deltoid, biceps, triceps, brachioradialis, wrist extensors, finger extensors and then APB, ADM and 1st DI (Figs 1.3 and 1.4). Test coordination and all the reflexes in the upper limbs. There are three common patterns of weakness:

- Weakness confined to APB is usually due to entrapment of the median nerve at the wrist within the carpal tunnel. If it is due to a lesion at the

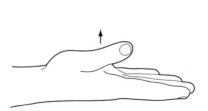

Figure 1.3 Abduction of the thumb.

Figure 1.4 Abduction of the fingers.

elbow, there will also be weakness of the deep flexors of the index finger and of flexor pollicis longus (Fig. 1.5). Ask the patient to make a fist; he or she may have the 'Benediction sign'[2] (Fig. 1.6a). Test power in the terminal phalanges of the index and thumb by getting the patient to form a figure 'O' with those digits (Fig. 1.6b). If those muscles are weak, the digits will assume the posture shown in Fig. 1.6c. Test whether there is a sensory loss in the distribution of the median nerve (Fig. 1.7).

- Weakness confined to ADM and 1st DI is usually due to an ulnar nerve lesion at the elbow (see Fig. 1.8). In severe cases there will also be weakness of the deep flexor of the little finger (see Fig. 1.9). Test for sensory loss in an ulnar distribution (Fig. 1.7). In the rare lesion of the deep palmar branch of the ulnar nerve, weakness is confined to abduction of the index and there is no sensory loss.
- Weakness of all three muscles has many causes, and it is not possible to make a definite diagnosis without performing a full neurological examination. In particular, it is important to check for:

  - Horner's syndrome
  - ptosis
  - facial weakness
  - wasting of the tongue
  - jaw jerk
  - wasting of the sternomastoids
  - wasting, weakness and reflex changes in all four limbs
  - sensory loss.

Certain patterns of neurological signs associated with wasting of the small muscles of the hand are characteristic:

2. Confusingly, the Benediction sign is also sometimes used to describe the posture in an ulnar nerve lesion where there is clawing of the ring and little fingers; in an ulnar nerve lesion the 'benediction' posture is seen at rest, in a median nerve lesion on attempting to make a fist.

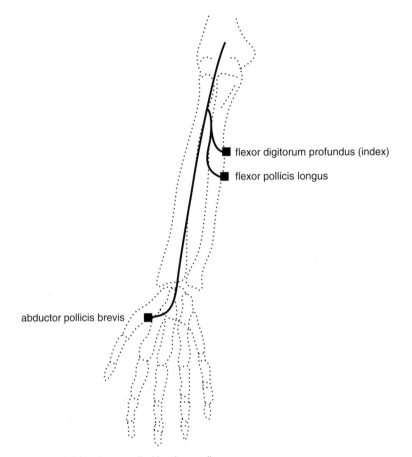

flexor digitorum profundus (index)

flexor pollicis longus

abductor pollicis brevis

Figure 1.5 Muscles supplied by the median nerve.

– Wasting confined to one hand and weakness of the finger extensors, finger flexors and triceps. The triceps reflex is absent, and there is sensory loss on the ulnar aspect of the forearm and hand (see Fig. 1.10). The patient has a C7, C8, T1 root or plexus lesion. If this is due to a cervical rib, there may also be a subclavian bruit and diminished pulses in the arm. In a Pancoast tumour there may be a Horner's syndrome, bovine cough, signs in the chest, lymphadenopathy and cachexia.

– 'Flail' arm with flaccid paralysis, wasting, areflexia and sensory loss confined to one arm. The commonest cause of this is avulsion of all the roots of the brachial plexus from C5–T1, often resulting from a motor-bike accident. Horner's syndrome is usually present.

(a)

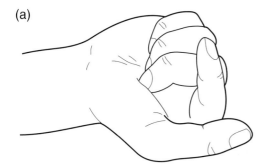

Figure 1.6 (a) 'Benediction' sign of a proximal lesion of the median nerve. (b) Testing flexor pollicis longus and the deep flexor of the index. (c) Posture adopted when flexor pollicis longus and the deep flexor of the index are weak.

(b)

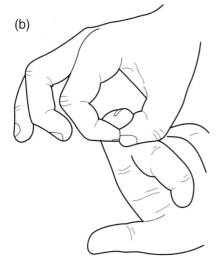

(c)

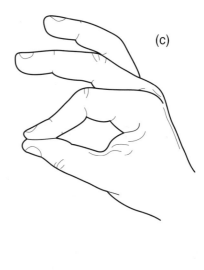

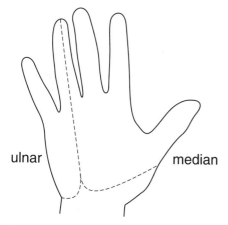

Figure 1.7 Sensory distribution of the median and ulnar nerves.

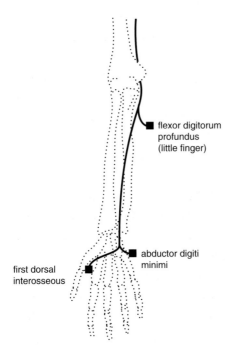

Figure 1.8 Muscles supplied by the ulnar nerve.

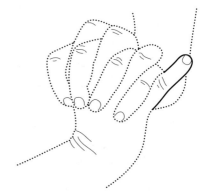

Figure 1.9 Weakness of flexor digitorum profundus of the little finger (proximal lesion of the ulnar nerve).

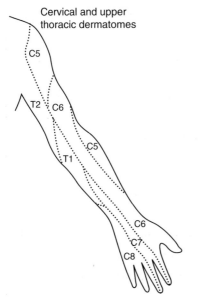

Figure 1.10 Dermatomes of the arm.

- Wasting of one hand, loss of reflexes in the arm and a dissociated sensory loss (loss of pain with preserved touch sensation) in a half-cape distribution on the same side. The hands may be swollen, cold and blue with the skin shiny, atrophic and scarred from previous unnoticed injuries. These are signs of an intrinsic lesion of the cervical and upper thoracic cord. Syringomyelia and tumours such as ependymoma should be considered. The signs may be bilateral.
- Wasting of both hands and spastic weakness of the legs. The patient has a C8,T1 cord lesion. There will usually be sensory loss to the appropriate level. Causes of this include tumour and trauma.
- Generalized muscle weakness and wasting, fasciculations, hyper-reflexia and normal sensation. The patient has motor neurone disease. Check the tongue for wasting and fasciculations (Box 1.1).
- Distal wasting and weakness of all four limbs, areflexia, and a glove and stocking sensory loss. The patient has a peripheral neuropathy.
- Distal wasting and weakness of all four limbs, hyporeflexia, baldness,

---

Box 1.1 Management issues in motor neurone disease (MND)

Investigations

- Electromyography (EMG) to confirm denervation (fasciculations, fibrillation potentials)
- Nerve conduction studies to exclude multifocal motor neuropathy with conduction block
- Magnetic resonance imaging (MRI) of brain and spinal cord: normal in MND
- Modified barium swallow to check for aspiration
- Respiratory function tests
- Exclude thyrotoxicosis

Treatment

- Supportive: nursing, social, end-of-life issues when disease is advanced
- Percutaneous endoscopic gastrostomy (PEG) feeding
- Nocturnal nasal continuous positive airway pressure (CPAP)
- Riluzole

ptosis and cataracts. The patient probably has dystrophia myotonica. Ask them to make a tight fist and then to open the fingers as rapidly as possible. If the fingers unfurl slowly, they have myotonia. Tap the thenar eminence. If the thumb slowly abducts and then falls back to its original position, they also have percussion myotonia.

Box 1.2 TIPS

- Candidates in examinations are sometimes asked whether wasting of the small muscles of the hand is likely to be due to cervical spondylosis. Cervical spondylosis is very common in older patients and, in most cases, is *not* the cause of marked muscle wasting in the hand; other causes should be considered.
- Generalized fasciculations are a key sign in the diagnosis of motor neurone disease. If you are considering this diagnosis, it is essential to disrobe the patient and to make a point of observing all parts of the musculature. Fasciculations are often best seen in triceps. Flickering movements of the calves and of the protruded tongue are common in normal individuals. They may also be seen in a generalized distribution in normal individuals. As a rule, fasciculations are rarely a matter of concern in the absence of muscle wasting, weakness and reflex changes.
- The commonest cause of coldness in a wasted hand is not vascular occlusion, but disuse.
- The commonest causes of wasting of the small muscles of the hands are old age and arthritis; in these conditions, muscle power in the wasted muscles is preserved.

Wrist drop

2

Inspection
Tone
Power, coordination and reflexes

Likely introduction: 'Weakness of the arm' or 'Examine the upper limbs'.

Wrist drop is due to weakness of extensor carpi radialis longus (supplied by C5/6 and the radial nerve) and extensor carpi ulnaris (supplied by C7/8 and the posterior interosseous branch of the radial nerve). It most commonly results from compression of the radial nerve in the spiral groove (Fig. 2.1). Causes include pressure ('Saturday night palsy') and diabetes. Wrist extension is also weak in lesions of the corticospinal tract. 04

Inspection

Wrist drop is seen when the arms are held out during the screening examination. In a posterior interosseous nerve lesion or C7/8 root lesion there will be radial deviation of the hand (Fig. 2.2). In a corticospinal lesion, the arm is slow to elevate and the elbow and wrist may remain a little flexed. Check for:

- bruising or scars, particularly over the spiral groove of the humerus in the posterior part of the upper arm (radial nerve palsy);
- facial asymmetry (hemiparesis); and/or
- muscle wasting, particularly in the extensor compartment of the forearm. Allow for the fact that the right forearm is usually thicker than the left in a right-handed person.

Tone

Tone in the upper limbs will be normal in a lesion of the peripheral nerve or roots and usually increased in a corticospinal lesion.

Power, coordination and reflexes

Test shoulder abduction, elbow flexion, elbow extension, brachioradialis, wrist extension, finger extension, finger flexion, finger abduction and thumb abduction. Test finger abduction with the hand resting on a surface (see Tips). Check coordination and reflexes in the upper limbs.

You are likely to find one of four patterns of weakness:

- Weakness of brachioradialis, wrist extension and finger extension. The patient has a radial nerve lesion. As triceps is normal and brachioradialis is weak, the lesion is likely to be in the spiral groove. The brachioradialis reflex is reduced or absent. There may be sensory loss in the region of the snuff box (Fig. 2.3).
- Weakness of finger extension with radial deviation of the wrist on attempted extension (signifying weakness of extensor carpi ulnaris). There is no sensory loss and reflexes are normal. The patient has a posterior interosseous nerve lesion (rare). This may result from entrapment of the nerve or be part of a mononeuritis multiplex (or simplex) of any cause (e.g. diabetes, collagen disease) (Box 2.1).
- Weakness of triceps and finger extensors and flexors; radial deviation of the wrist on attempted extension. The triceps reflex is reduced or absent. The patient has a C7/8 root or plexus lesion. These signs may be seen in cervical spondylosis or a brachial plexus injury.
- Generalized weakness of the muscles of the upper limb which is most marked in deltoid, triceps, wrist extension and finger extension. The patient has a corticospinal lesion. Tone and reflexes are likely to be increased. Look for evidence of weakness in the face and leg on the same side (hemiparesis).

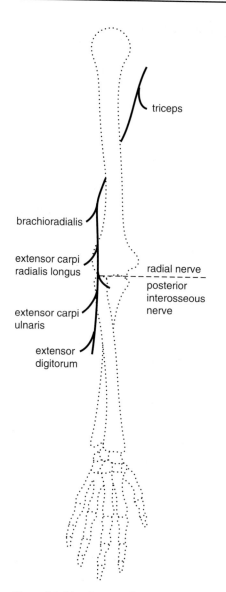

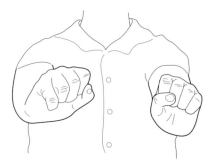

Figure 2.2 Radial deviation in a right posterior interosseous nerve lesion.

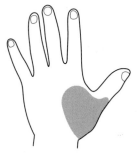

Figure 2.3 Sensory loss over the snuffbox in a radial nerve lesion.

triceps

brachioradialis

extensor carpi radialis longus

radial nerve

posterior interosseous nerve

extensor carpi ulnaris

extensor digitorum

Figure 2.1 Muscles supplied by the radial nerve.

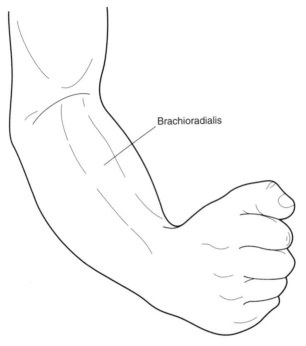

Brachioradialis

Figure 2.4 Brachioradialis.

Box 2.1 Management issues in mononeuritis multiplex

Investigations

- Nerve conduction studies
- Electromyography (EMG) to confirm denervation
- Cerebrospinal fluid (CSF) protein in demyelinating neuropathy
- Blood tests might include: fasting glucose, glucose tolerance test, anti-GM1 and GQ1b antibodies, and screening for HIV, hepatitis C (cryoglobulins), *Campylobacter*, vasculitis (ANA, ENA, ANCA), and sarcoidosis (serum calcium, alkaline phosphatase and angiotensin-converting enzyme)

Treatment

- Underlying cause: e.g. diabetes
- Supportive: foot splint for foot drop

Box 2.2 TIPS

- It is almost impossible to abduct the fingers when they are flexed at the metocarpophalangeal joints. Try it yourself. In wrist drop, the fingers are also flexed and it is essential, therefore, for you to correct this before asking the patient to attempt to perform finger abduction. This is best done by resting the hand in the prone position on a flat surface.
- Brachioradialis is the key muscle to test in a suspected radial nerve palsy (Fig. 2.4).

Proximal weakness of the arm(s)

3

Inspection
Tone
Power, coordination and reflexes

Likely introduction: 'Weakness of the arm(s)' or 'Perform a motor examination on this patient's upper limbs'.

The proximal muscles of the upper limb which are routinely tested are:

- deltoid: shoulder abduction; axillary nerve; C5/6 roots
- biceps: elbow flexion; musculocutaneous nerve; C5/6 roots
- triceps: elbow extension; radial nerve; C7/8 roots
- brachioradialis: elbow flexion with the thumb pointing to the shoulder; radial nerve; C5/6 roots

Under some circumstances it is useful to test:

- supraspinatus: first 20° of shoulder abduction; suprascapular nerve; C5/6 roots
- infraspinatus: external rotation at the shoulder; suprascapular nerve; C5/6 roots
- trapezius: shoulder elevation; spinal accessory nerve (superior portion); C3/4 (inferior portion)
- serratus anterior: scapular fixation and rotation; long thoracic nerve; C5/6/7

Deltoid can only function effectively if the scapula is firmly anchored by trapezius and serratus anterior (Fig. 3.1). Rotation of the scapula increases the range of abduction possible at the shoulder.

Unilateral weakness confined to the proximal upper limb is usually due to a lesion of the cervical roots, brachial plexus or peripheral nerves. In

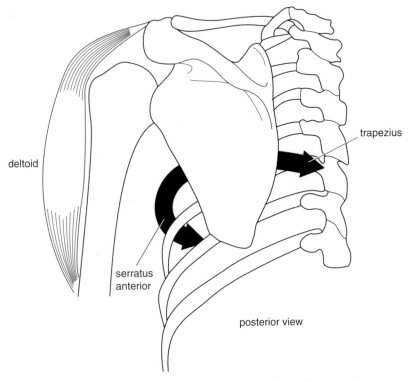

Figure 3.1 Mode of action of trapezius and serratus anterior on the scapula.

corticospinal lesions all the extensors of the upper limb, proximal and distal, are weak. Bilateral proximal weakness of the upper limbs is likely to be due to a myopathy (Box 3.1).

Inspection

Remove all garments from the patient's trunk and upper limbs and look for the following:

- **Skin.** A purple ('heliotrope') rash around the eyes and on the cheeks and a scaly erythema at the base of the finger nails and on the elbows and knees are features of dermatomyositis.
- **Joints.** Look for subluxation of the humerus (Fig. 3.2).
- **Wasting.** This is most obvious in deltoid. Look at the shoulder from the back as well as the front or you may miss winging of the scapula.

Box 3.1 Management issues in chronic myopathy

Investigations

- Electromyography (EMG) to confirm myopathic changes
- Muscle biopsy to confirm inflammatory or other specific changes
- Blood tests might include: erythrocyte sedimentation rate (ESR), C-reactive protein (CRP), creatine phosphokinase (CPK), auto-immune screen

Treatment

- Underlying cause: immunosuppression, steroids
- Supportive: physiotherapy

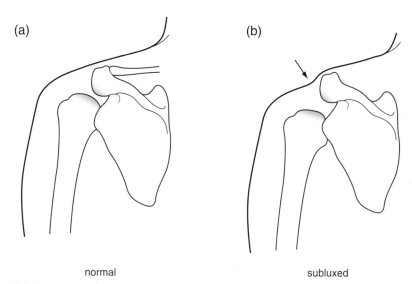

(a) (b)

normal subluxed

Figure 3.2 (a) Profile of normal shoulder joint. (b) Profile of shoulder in downward subluxation of the humerus.

- **Face.** This may provide important clues: unilateral ptosis (Horner's syndrome with an avulsion injury of the cervical roots and T1); bilateral ptosis (dystrophia myotonica, myasthenia gravis, myopathy); facial droop (as part of a hemiparesis).
- **Fasciculations.** Motor neurone disease.

Tone

This will be normal in disorders of the peripheral nerves or muscle and may be increased in a corticospinal lesion.

Power, coordination and reflexes

Test shoulder abduction, elbow flexion and extension, brachioradialis, wrist extension and flexion and finger extension, flexion and abduction. Check coordination and reflexes in the upper limbs. There are a number of characteristic patterns of weakness, each associated with other signs:

- Weakness confined to deltoid. This cannot be a C5/6 root lesion for biceps and brachioradialis are spared (Fig. 3.3). Make certain that the scapula does not move as the arm gives way when shoulder abduction is tested. If it does not, the patient has an axillary nerve lesion. Reflexes will be normal. There may be an area of sensory loss over the deltoid.
- Weakness of deltoid, biceps and brachioradialis, with normal power in the other muscles tested so far. This is a C5/6 cord, root or plexus lesion. To determine the level of the lesion, other signs need to be considered:

  - C5/6 cord lesion. Here, the reflexes at the level of the lesion – biceps and brachioradialis – are absent while those below that level – triceps and the lower limb reflexes – are increased. The vibration caused by tapping the radius to elicit the brachioradialis reflex may cause the fingers to flex; the finger flexors arise below the site of the lesion (at C7/8) and are therefore more easily excited. Some flexion is common in normal individuals, but if flexion of the fingers occurs without contraction of the brachioradialis in response to tapping of the radius (the 'inverted supinator' reflex) a C5/6 cord lesion is probably present. Test tone and power in the lower limbs and look for a sensory level at C5.
  - C5/6 root or plexus lesion. Here, the biceps and brachioradialis reflexes are absent but the triceps reflex and leg reflexes are normal. The point at which these nerves have been damaged is determined by testing muscles, also supplied by the C5/6 roots, in the order in which they arise (Fig. 3.3). Thus, a very proximal lesion will involve all the C5/6 muscles. Further

05

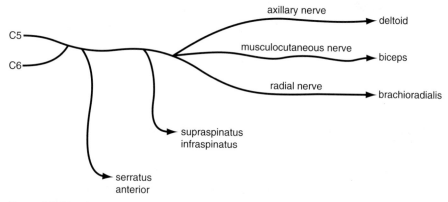

Figure 3.3 Muscles supplied by C5 and C6.

down, serratus anterior is spared and further down still, supraspinatus and infraspinatus will be spared. In a C5/6 root or plexus lesion there is likely to be sensory loss in the same dermatomes (see Fig. 1.10).

- Weakness of all the muscles of one arm with:

  - Absence of reflexes in the arm. If the other limbs are normal the patient probably has a brachial plexus lesion. Check for a Horner's syndrome and a C5–T1 sensory loss. If there is a dissociated sensory loss consider intrinsic cord lesions such as syringomyelia.
  - Hyper-reflexia. Use your screening tests on the face and legs to determine whether this is part of a hemiparesis. With a right hemiparesis check for aphasia (see below). With a left hemiparesis, test for signs of neglect (sensory and visual), constructional apraxia and dressing apraxia.

- Weakness of the proximal muscles of both arms. This is likely to be due to a disorder of muscle (myopathy) or neuromuscular junction. Test power and reflexes in the lower limbs. There are several characteristic patterns of signs:

  - Weakness of all the proximal muscles of the arms and legs. Reflexes are normal or reduced. Sensation is normal. Consider polymyositis, particularly in an older person, if there is muscle tenderness on palpation or if there is a skin rash (dermatomyositis). Myasthenia gravis is also a possibility. Check for fatigability by repeatedly pressing down on the arms held abducted and flexed at the elbows. Test for weakness of neck flexion (see Tips).

- Selective weakness and wasting of the proximal muscles of the arms and legs. Here, certain muscles are almost completely wasted while their neighbour, perhaps with the same root supply, is normal. Thus, brachioradialis (C5/6) may be wasted while deltoid (also C5/6) is spared. There may be winging of the scapula. These are the findings of muscular dystrophy, spinal muscular atrophy and inclusion body myositis (rare in practice, common in examinations!). Test facial movements and eye closure. The patient could be of any age but is more likely to be young. If the reflexes are lost you should consider spinal muscular atrophy.

- Weakness of the muscles which fixate the scapula usually becomes apparent during testing of deltoid. You find weakness of shoulder abduction, but on careful inspection and palpation it becomes clear that you are not 'breaking' deltoid, rather, you are forcing the scapula to rotate. The patient has weakness of trapezius, serratus anterior or both. Check the following:

  - Note the position of the shoulders. In weakness of trapezius, one shoulder will be lower than the other. Compare the muscle bulk of trapezius on the two sides. Wasting of trapezius is often visible and palpable.
  - Compare the sternomastoids on both sides. The accessory nerve supplies both trapezius and sternomatoid.
  - Ask the patient to push the extended arms against the wall. The vertebral border of the scapula lifts away from the thorax ('wings') if there is weakness of serratus anterior. Isolated weakness of serratus anterior is quite common. It follows injury to the long thoracic nerve by, for example, cervical gland biopsy. It is also one manifestation of neuralgic amyotrophy.

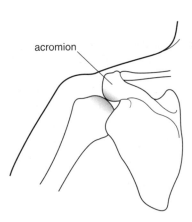

acromion

Figure 3.4 Restriction of abduction of the humerus by the acromion in upward subluxation associated with a rotator cuff tear.

Box 3.2 TIPS

- Weakness of shoulder abduction can be due to weakness of deltoid or failure of serratus anterior and trapezius to fixate the scapula. Feel the tip of the scapula with one hand as you test shoulder abduction with the other hand. If the scapula moves, the problem is at least in part due to weakness of serratus anterior or trapezius. The strength of deltoid can be tested separately by manually fixating the scapula as you test shoulder abduction.

- Brachioradialis is one of the most useful muscles to test. It is important in diagnosing C5/6 root lesions and in localizing the site of a radial nerve lesion. It is often selectively wasted in muscular dystrophy. Both biceps and brachioradialis flex the elbow; weakness of brachioradialis cannot be demonstrated by overcoming elbow flexion, for biceps is more than adequate for this task. Weakness in brachioradialis is detected by observing and feeling the muscle when elbow flexion is resisted with the forearm midway between pronation and supination (see Fig. 2.5): "Pull your thumb towards your nose". A weak brachioradialis remains soft during this procedure or fails to contract at all.

- Always test for weakness of neck flexion when you find proximal weakness of the arms. This is characteristically present in myopathies and myasthenia gravis.

- Patients with rotator cuff injuries of the shoulder can be confusing. When asked to abduct the shoulder they are only able to do so to a limited extent, and you may mistakenly diagnose an axillary nerve lesion. The following features should make you consider this possibility:

  - while abduction is limited, forward flexion of the elbow is normal. The reason for this is that the humerus subluxes upwards when the rotator cuff is ruptured and the coracoid bone prevents full abduction (Fig. 3.4).
  - the long head of biceps is ruptured, causing the biceps to 'bunch up' in elbow flexion.
  - on attempted abduction the shoulder is elevated, giving it a characteristic shrugging appearance.
  - the range of passive movement of the shoulder is limited and sometimes painful.

Proximal weakness of the leg(s)

4

Inspection
Tone
Power, coordination and reflexes

Likely introduction: 'Difficulty walking', or 'Examine the motor system in the lower limbs'.

The proximal muscles of the legs which are routinely tested are:

- Iliopsoas: hip flexion; femoral nerve; L1/2/3 roots.
- Quadriceps: knee extension; femoral nerve; L2/3/4 roots.
- Gluteus maximus: hip extension; inferior gluteal nerve; L5, S1/2 roots.
- Hamstrings: knee flexion; sciatic nerve; L5, S1/2 roots.
- Hip adductors: obturator nerve; L2/3/4.

Weakness which is confined to the proximal muscles of the legs is usually due to a disorder of muscle (e.g. myopathy) or neuromuscular junction (e.g. myasthenia gravis). Weakness of proximal and distal muscles is seen in Guillain–Barré[1] syndrome and motor neurone disease. Unilateral proximal weakness is often due to a femoral nerve lesion.

Inspection

- Observe the gait. This may be:

- waddling, with exaggerated shoulder sway, in any cause of proximal weakness or in hip joint disorders.

---

1. *Georges Guillain, French neurologist at the Salpetriere, Paris (1876–1961); JA Barré, French neurologist (1880–1967).*

- antalgic, the stride when weight bearing on the painful side is faster and shorter than on the good side.
- hemiparetic (see section on gait).

- Ask the patient to rise from a crouching position. Patients with proximal weakness of the lower limbs cannot get up. Children with muscular dystrophy may 'climb up' themselves, using their arms as levers (Gowers'[2] sign).
- Look for wasting in quadriceps. This is most obvious with the patient standing. You may wish to compare the circumference of the thighs at a defined distance above the knee but it is difficult to do this accurately.
- Look for fasciculations.
- Check the lower spine for scars and the buttocks for wasting.
- Note whether the hip remains flexed when the patient lies down: this may signify disease of the hip joint.

Tone

Test tone in the lower limbs. This will be normal in lesions of the peripheral nerves and muscles and increased in corticospinal lesions. Internally and externally rotating the hip may reveal pain and limitation of movement due to hip disease.

Power, coordination and reflexes

Test hip flexion and extension, knee flexion and extension, ankle dorsiflexion and plantar flexion, eversion and inversion. Ask the patient to run the heel up and down the shin on each leg in turn. Test the knee, ankle and plantar reflexes.

You are likely to find one of the following patterns of abnormality:

- Weakness of iliopsoas and weakness and wasting of quadriceps. The knee jerk is reduced or absent. Power in the hip adductors is normal (see Tips). The patient has a femoral nerve lesion (Fig. 4.1). There may also

2. Sir William Gowers, Queen Square neurologist, author of Diseases of the Nervous System, the 'Bible' for neurologists for many years (1845–1915)

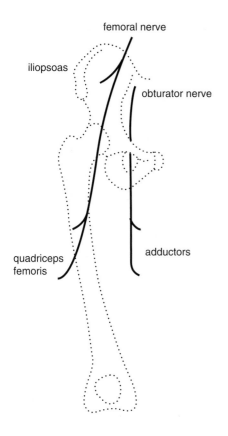

femoral nerve

iliopsoas

obturator nerve

quadriceps
femoris

adductors

Figure 4.1 Muscles supplied by the femoral and obturator nerves.

be sensory impairment over the thigh and medial aspect of the shin. An important cause of a painful femoral nerve lesion is adult-onset diabetes mellitus (diabetic amyotrophy). Haemorrhage into the psoas as a result of anticoagualant therapy and traction during hip surgery are other causes.

- Weakness of iliopsoas, quadriceps and hip adductors. The knee jerk is reduced or absent. The patient has an L2/3/4 root or plexus lesion. There is likely to be sensory loss in the equivalent dermatomes. If the lesion involves the cauda equina within the vertebral canal, both legs are likely to be involved. The most likely cause is a tumour, either primary or secondary. Prolapse of an intervertebral disc is uncommon at this spinal level. There are many causes of a femoral plexus lesion including pelvic malignancy, obstetric injury and neuralgic amyotrophy.

- Weakness of one leg, most marked in hip flexion, knee flexion, ankle dorsiflexion and eversion. Tone and reflexes are increased. The patient has a corticospinal lesion. Perform screening tests on the face and arm looking for evidence of a hemiparesis.
- Weakness of both legs, most marked in hip flexion, knee flexion, ankle dorsiflexion and eversion. Tone and reflexes are increased. The patient has a paraparesis. The lesion is likely to be in the spinal cord. Look for a motor and sensory level.
- Diffuse weakness of the proximal muscles of both legs. Check power and reflexes in the upper limbs. If there is also proximal weakness of the arms your assessment will largely hinge on the reflex findings:

  - Reflexes are preserved or reduced. Consider a myopathy (e.g. muscular dystrophy or polymyositis) or myasthenia gravis (check for fatigability).
  - Reflexes are lost. Consider spinal muscular atrophy or myasthenic syndrome (Eaton–Lambert[3] syndrome). The reflexes are also lost in Guillain–Barré syndrome, but here there is likely to be distal as well as proximal weakness.
  - Reflexes are increased. Consider motor neurone disease (check for fasciculations; wasting and fasciculation of the tongue; sensation) or causes of a quadriparesis such as multilacunar state (check gait, jaw jerk, speech, mental state) or cervical myelopathy (normal cranial nerves; loss of some reflexes in the arms, depending on the level).

- Other patterns of proximal weakness are much less common. Weakness confined to hip adduction is seen with obturator nerve lesions (obstetric injury). Selective lesions of the superior gluteal nerve (which supplies gluteus medius and minimus and tensor fasciae latae) and of the inferior gluteal nerve (which supplies gluteus maximus) are very uncommon indeed. Sciatic nerve lesions are a cause of distal weakness of the leg, with or without weakness of hamstrings.

---

3. LM Eaton, American neurologist at the Mayo Clinic (1905–1958).

Box 4.1 TIPS

- Arthritis of the hip or knee can cause wasting and weakness of quadriceps and diminution or loss of the knee jerk.
- Pain and wasting of quadriceps can be the presenting symptom of adult-onset diabetes mellitus.
- Weakness and wasting of quadriceps can be due to a femoral nerve lesion or an L2/3/4 root (or plexus) lesion. To distinguish between the two, you need to test a muscle which has the same root but a different nerve supply. The hip adductors fulfil this requirement being supplied by L2/3/4 but via the obturator nerve.

Foot drop

5

| Inspection |
| Tone |
| Power, coordination and reflexes |

Likely introduction: 'Difficulty in walking' or 'Examine the motor system in the lower limbs'.

Foot drop is due to weakness of tibialis anterior, a muscle supplied by the common peroneal nerve and L4/5 roots. The common peroneal nerve also supplies the peroneal muscles which evert the foot; the L4/5 roots also supply tibialis posterior which inverts the foot. Weakness of tibialis anterior can result from lesions of the corticospinal tract as well as from lesions of the peripheral nerves or roots.

Inspection

- **Gait.** Get the patient to walk in an open space where the arms can swing freely. The foot is plantar-flexed and inverted and the gait high-stepping in a common peroneal nerve lesion. In a corticospinal lesion, the foot is also inverted but the leg swings in an arc, allowing the toe to clear the ground (circumduction). In a patient with a stroke, the arm may fail to swing. Ask the patient to stand on their toes and then their heels.
- **Wasting.** Remove all clothing from the patient's lower limbs after checking that they are wearing an undergarment. Observe the skin, joints and posture and look for wasting. Wasting is most obvious in tibialis anterior in a common peroneal nerve lesion. This is seen as a loss of the normal convexity lateral to the ridge of the tibia, and is easily missed in a patient lying on a couch, if the knees are not lifted. If the calf muscles are also wasted, a number of conditions need to be considered (see below).

- **Pes cavus** (Fig. 5.1). This sign tells you that the lesion is long-standing. Causes include Charcot–Marie–Tooth[1] disease, Friedreich's[2] ataxia and spina bifida.
- **Fasciculations.**
- **The lower spine.** This should be inspected for evidence of spina bifida (lipoma or tuft of hair), spinal deformity or previous surgery.
- Ask the patient to lie on the couch and fully dorsiflex both feet. This is useful for detecting mild unilateral footdrop.
- Check the legs for scars or bruises, particularly over the head of the fibula in a patient with unilateral foot drop.

Tone

Test tone at the knees and look for clonus at the ankles in both legs. Tone is normal in peripheral nerve and root lesions and increased in lesions of the corticospinal tract.

Power, coordination and reflexes

Check hip flexion and extension, knee flexion and extension, ankle dorsiflexion, plantar flexion, and inversion and eversion in both legs. Get the patient to run each heel in turn up and down the shin. Test the knee, ankle and plantar reflexes. There are four common patterns of weakness:

- Weakness of dorsiflexion and eversion. The patient has a common peroneal nerve lesion (Fig. 5.2), and there will also be weakness of extensor hallucis longus. Reflexes in the leg will be normal, and there may be the typical sensory loss (Fig. 5.3). Look for scars or bruising over the head of the fibula. In the rare lesion of the deep peroneal nerve, eversion is normal and the area of sensory loss very small (Fig. 5.4).
- Weakness of dorsiflexion, eversion and inversion. The patient has an L4/5 root or plexus lesion. Causes of this include a prolapsed intervertebral disc, tumour of the cauda equina and obstetric injury to the lumbo-sacral trunk (Fig. 5.5). Reflexes in the leg are likely to be normal. There may also

---

1. *Jean-Martin Charcot, French neurologist at the Salpetriere, Paris one of the founders of the discipline of neurology (1825–1893); Pierre Marie, French neurologist (1853–1940); Howard Henry Tooth, Queen Square neurologist (1856–1926).*
2. *Nikolaus Friedreich, German pathologist and physician (1825–1882).*

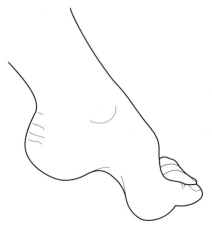

Figure 5.1 Pes cavus.

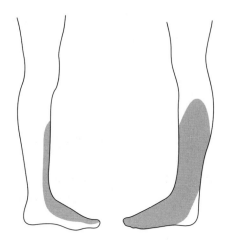

Figure 5.3 Sensory loss in a common peroneal nerve lesion.

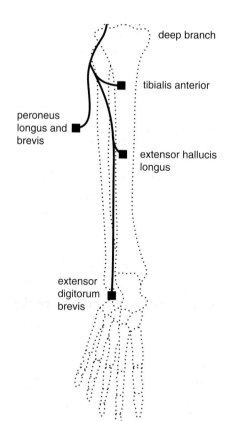

deep branch

tibialis anterior

peroneus longus and brevis

extensor hallucis longus

extensor digitorum brevis

Figure 5.2 Muscles supplied by the common peroneal nerve).

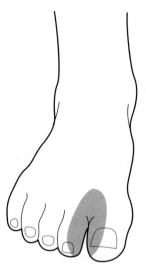

Figure 5.4 Sensory loss in a lesion of the deep branch of the common peroneal nerve.

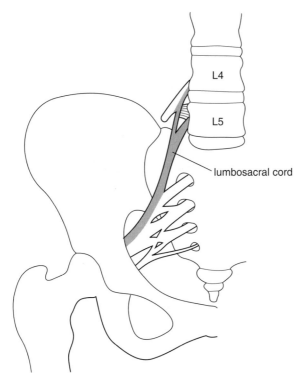

L4

L5

lumbosacral cord

Figure 5.5 The lumbosacral cord arising from the L4, L5 roots.

be weakness of hip abduction and sensory symptoms or signs in the L4/5 dermatomes (Fig. 5.6).

- Weakness of all movements of the foot with normal power at the knee and hip. There are several possibilities:

  - Peripheral neuropathy (with distal weakness of both legs, areflexia and glove and stocking sensory loss) (Box 5.1).
  - Sciatic nerve lesion (rare) due to pressure, trauma, vasculitis or tumour (with loss of the ankle jerk, extensive sensory loss and, depending on the site of the lesion, weakness of the hamstrings).
  - Root or plexus lesion (with loss of the ankle jerk and anal reflex, saddle anaesthesia (Fig. 5.7) and urinary incontinence). The cauda equina may be involved by tumour or prolapsed disc, the plexus by tumour or trauma.
  - Anterior horn cell disease due to motor neurone disease (with wasting, fasciculation, hyper-reflexia and normal sensation).

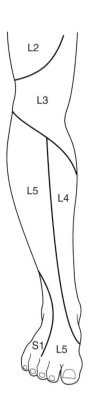

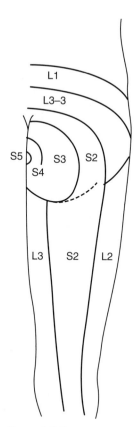

Figure 5.6 Dermatomes of the lower leg.

Figure 5.7 Dermatomes of the buttock.

- Weakness of hip flexion, knee flexion, dorsiflexion and eversion. Tone in the leg is increased and the reflexes are brisk. The patient has a lesion of the corticospinal tract. The following patterns of signs are useful in localizing the site of the lesion:

- Both legs are weak (paraparesis). This is usually due to a spinal cord lesion. If this is in the thoracic cord (e.g. due to a meningioma), the arms will be spared and there will be a sensory level on the trunk. If it is due to a cervical cord lesion, there will be loss of reflexes at the appropriate level (C5/6: biceps and brachioradialis; C7/8: triceps). Parasagittal tumours pressing on the motor strips of the cerebral hemispheres is a rare cause of weakness of both legs.

- One leg is weak. Possibilities include: (i) Brown-Séquard[3] syndrome:

3. *Charles Edouard Brown–Séquard, Mauritian-born neurologist who practised at Queen Square and later Paris (1817–1894).*

Box 5.1 Management issues in chronic peripheral neuropathy.

Investigations

- Nerve conduction studies to determine if it is axonal or demyelinating
- Electromyography (EMG) to confirm denervation
- Nerve biopsy
- Cerebrospinal fluid (CSF) protein (raised in inflammatory demyelinating neuropathy)
- Blood tests
- Fasting glucose, glucose tolerance test
- Vitamin B_{12}, folate
- Antinuclear antibody (ANA), extractable nuclear antigens (ENA), anti-neutrophil cytoplasmic autoantibodies (ANCA) for vasculitis

Treatment

- Underlying cause: e.g. diabetes, vitamin B_{12}
- Supportive: physiotherapy, foot splint for foot drop
- Plasma exchange/steroids/immunosuppression for chronic relapsing demyelinating neuropathies
- Neuropathic pain: valproate, amitryptyline, gabapentin

---

check for dissociated sensory loss in the other leg (see Tips); and (ii) anterior cerebral artery occlusion: check for a grasp reflex in the hand on the same side. If it is the right leg which is weak, the patient may be aphasic.

- The arm and leg are weak on the same side (hemiparesis). The lesion is likely to be above the cervical cord. The commonest causes are a stroke or tumour in the contralateral cerebral hemisphere.

Box 5.2 TIPS

- Pes cavus is a useful sign as long as it is not overdiagnosed. It is not enough to have a high arch. There should also be clawing of the toes and the foot should be thick (see Fig. 5.1). These signs are most apparent when the foot is dependent.

- In testing eversion and inversion of the foot, prevent the patient from rotating the hip by immobilizing the shin with one hand. With the other hand, move the foot into the required position, for example into the fully inverted position, and ask them to hold it there. Then attempt to evert the foot.

- In any patient with absent ankle jerks, it is important to test buttock sensation, as in lesions of the cauda equina sensation elsewhere may be normal.

- Absence of the ankle jerk is a key sign. Take time to put the patient at ease. Use the Jendrassik[4] manoeuvre. Sometimes the reflex can be obtained more readily by tapping the sole of the foot than by tapping the Achilles tendon. If you are still in doubt, ask the patient to kneel on a chair and tap the tendon while gently dorsiflexing the foot.

- Remember: the spinal cord ends at the second lumbar vertebra. Lesions above this will cause increased tone and reflexes, below it decreased tone and areflexia.

- Selective nerve lesions often occur in the setting of a generalized peripheral neuropathy. In diabetes, for example, a patient may have a foot drop with the typical distribution of weakness of a common peroneal nerve lesion. In addition, the ankle jerk may be lost due to an underlying peripheral neuropathy. Peripheral neuropathy predisposes nerves to pressure palsy.

- A sign of particular importance is dissociated sensory loss where the patient can feel the lightest touch in the affected area but is unable to distinguish one end of a pin from the other. Selective involvement of the pain pathways is a feature of syringomyelia, hemi-cord lesions (Brown–Séquard syndrome) and the lateral medullary syndrome.

4. E. Jendrassik, Hungarian neurologist (1858–1921).

- Wasting of extensor digitorum brevis is often found in peripheral neuropathies and in lesions of the common peroneal nerve. In a normal subject, the muscle stands out like a grape when the toes are dorsiflexed against resistance.
- Weakness of extension of the great toe may be the only motor sign of an L5 root lesion in a patient with sciatica.
- Spasticity of the legs (increased tone, hyper-reflexia, clonus) with well-preserved power (and no sensory loss or bladder involvement) is the characteristic finding in hereditary spastic paraplegia (rare in practice, common in examinations). Hydrocephalus may also cause spasticity of the legs.

Gait disturbance

6

Likely introduction: 'Difficulty in walking' or 'Examine the gait'.

The observation of gait is probably the single most useful part of the neurological examination. It provides you with an opportunity to see the patient as a whole. Muscle weakness, impairment of balance, sensory loss, involuntary movements, abnormalities of posture, even mood disturbance and dementia may all leave a distinctive imprint on the way we walk. Gait is sadly neglected, yet the extra few moments taken to observe it are rarely wasted. In some diseases, such as Parkinson's disease,[1] the gait is so distinctive that the diagnosis is clear as the patient walks into the room. To benefit from observing gait, you must train your eye to take a note of a number of key features (listed below). In this chapter, a number of gaits are described and illustrated on video in the accompanying CD.

In the setting of a short case, the assessment of gait itself will, of necessity, be brief. It serves as a pointer to the aspects of the neurological examination on which you should focus. The more you can learn from the gait, the more likely you are to direct the rest of the examination appropriately.

Observation

- Never attempt to assess gait in a confined space such as a small examination room with a couch in it. You will not be able to judge stride length or arm swing under these conditions. Get the patient to walk in an open corridor.

---

1. James Parkinson, London physician and palaeontologist (1755–1824).

- Don't stand too close. Candidates often hover anxiously beside the patient. If you are afraid that the patient will fall, ask for a nurse to walk with the patient.
- Don't base your assessment on a couple of strides. Get the patient to walk about 10 metres, turn and come back. In a difficult case you may want to repeat this.
- Make particular note of the following (Fig. 6.1):

  - Posture of the head, trunk and limbs
  - Arm swing
  - Stride length
  - Base or stance (Fig. 6.2)
  - Involuntary movements

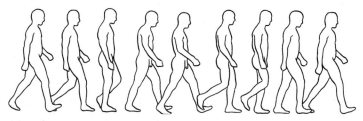

Figure 6.1 Normal gait (from the side).

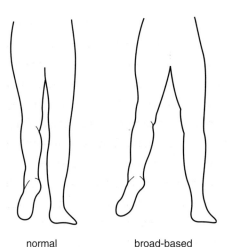

normal   broad-based

Figure 6.2 Normal and broad-based gait (from behind).

- Ask the patient to stand on their toes. This is a sensitive test for weakness in gastrocnemius-soleus.
- Ask the patient to stand on their heels. Failure to do this will confirm the presence of footdrop.
- Do the Romberg test (see Tips).
- If the patient appears to be parkinsonian, check the righting reflex (see below).

Further assessment

There are a number of distinctive patterns of gait disturbance:

- One foot is lifted higher than the other during each stride. The affected foot hangs downwards while it is elevated. The patient has a *high-stepping gait* due to unilateral foot drop. This is usually caused by a common peroneal nerve lesion (see section on 'Foot drop'). In such a case, the patient will be able to walk on their toes but not on their heel, on the affected side.

  08

- Both feet are lifted higher than normal and may produce a slapping sound as they hit the ground. This type of high-stepping gait is most commonly due to bilateral foot drop due, for example, to a peripheral neuropathy such as Charcot–Marie–Tooth disease. Motor neurone disease is another cause. Such a patient will have difficulty walking on their toes or heels.

  10

- A similar high-stepping gait is seen where there is impairment of sensation in the feet (sensory ataxia). The gait is wide-based and the patient watches the ground and their feet intently. Test for Romberg's[2] sign (see Tips). Place the patient between you and the wall, and ask them to put their feet together and to shut their eyes. In such a case, the patient may start to fall, without making any apparent attempt to stop themselves. You, of course, must prevent them from falling, but it may be difficult if the patient is very large. Under these circumstances ask for assistance or explain to the examiners why you are not going to do the test. You will need to test position sense in the feet. Causes of sensory ataxia include sensory neuropathy, tabes dorsalis, spinocerebellar degeneration, subacute combined degeneration of the cord and multiple sclerosis.

2. *Moritz Heinrich Romberg, German physician, author of one of the first textbooks in neurology (1795–1873)*

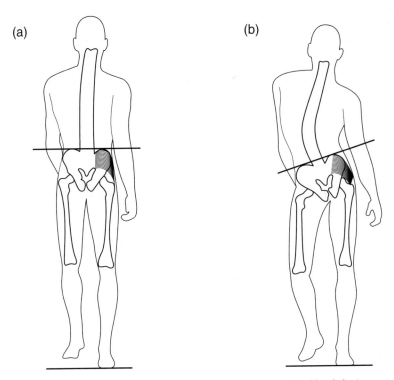

Figure 6.3 (a) Normal Trendelenburg test; (b) weakness of right hip abductors.

- The shoulders sway from side to side in an exaggerated manner with each stride. The patient appears to be lifting the foot off the ground, not only by flexing the hip and knee but also by tilting the trunk. This is a *waddling gait*. It signifies weakness of hip abduction and can be demonstrated using Trendelenburg's[3] test (Fig. 6.3a,b). When the left foot is lifted off the ground, the pelvis is normally prevented from tilting downwards on the left side by the action of the right hip abductors. When these are weak, the buttock is seen to sag. It may take a number of seconds before this occurs. Weakness of hip abduction can result from muscle pathology, or from disturbance of the normal fulcrum provided by the hip joint. You will need to test proximal muscle power and put the hips through a full range of movements. A waddling gait in a child is likely to be due to muscular dystrophy or congenital dislocation of the hips. In an adult, consider a myopathy and osteoarthritis of the hips.

3. Friedrich Trendelenburg, German surgeon (1844–1924).

- One leg is held stiffly, and describes an arc around the other leg with each stride (circumduction). The foot scrapes the ground. The arm on the same side does not swing and is flexed at the elbow. This is a *hemiparetic gait*. There may be obvious facial weakness. You will need to test tone, power and reflexes in the limbs. The most common cause in an adult is stroke (Box 6.1).

Box 6.1 Management issues in stroke.

Investigations

- Computed tomography (CT) initially to exclude haemorrhage
- Blood tests might include: cholesterol, full blood picture (FBP) and platelets
- Cardiac:

  - Electrocardiography
  - Echocardiography

- MRI with diffusion-weighted imaging to localize site of recent lesion(s)
- Doppler studies of neck vessels in strokes in carotid territory
- Fat suppression MRI of neck in suspected dissection (younger patients, history of trauma, painful Horner's syndrome)
- Pro-thrombotic screening (protein C and S, anti-phospholipid a/b in younger patients, history of deep vein thrombosis (DVT), miscarriages)

Treatment

- Antiplatelet agents for large-vessel atheroma
- Warfarin for cardioembolic strokes
- Carotid endarterectomy for symptomatic severe carotid stenosis
- Thrombolysis
- DVT prophylaxis
- Rehabilitation

- Both legs are held stiffly and show circumduction. The steps are short and slow, as though the patient is wading through water. The feet are inverted and may cross ('scissor'). This is a spastic paraparetic or *scissoring gait*. It is seen in its most florid form in longstanding disorders such as cerebral palsy and hereditary spastic paraplegia. Scissoring is less of a feature when paraparesis is acquired later in life, for example in association with cervical spondylosis or multiple sclerosis.

- The patient fails to swing one arm as they walk. The gait is otherwise normal. The patient may have early Parkinson's disease (check for tremor, rigidity and akinesia). Test shoulder joint mobility; frozen shoulder can also interfere with the arm swing. Patients who have made an otherwise good recovery from stroke may also have reduced arm swing.

- The patient is flexed at the neck, elbows, hips and knees. The arms fail to swing. Steps are small and shuffling. Several steps are taken in turning. The base is normal. This is a *Parkinsonian gait*. Other features which may be present include: hand tremor; hurrying (festination); a tendency to run forwards (propulsion) or backwards (retropulsion); getting suddenly stuck and unable to go on, particularly when changing direction or going through a doorway (freezing).

  - Patients with advanced Parkinson's disease often have an impaired righting reflex. This is tested by using the Pull test: stand behind the patient, warn them that you are going to give their shoulders a tug, and then do so. If balance is normal, the patient steps back. In mild impairment the patient staggers, but then recovers. In severe cases, the patient runs backwards uncontrollably (i.e. develops retropulsion) or begins to fall. As with Romberg's test, be careful with large patients. You are less likely to end up on the floor with the patient if you stand with your back close to the wall as you do the test.

- The posture is upright, but the arms fail to swing and the steps are small and shuffling. Several steps are taken in turning. The appearance is similar to Parkinson's disease with one important difference: it is broad-based. This is called '*marche à petits pas*' (from the French, 'gait with small steps') and is seen particularly in multi-lacunar states (associated with emotional lability, dementia, generalized hyper-reflexia, positive jaw-jerk) and normal pressure hydrocephalus (associated with cognitive impairment and incontinence of urine).

- The gait is broad-based, with unsteady irregular steps. There is a tendency to veer to one side or the other and to stagger on turning. These are the features of a cerebellar or *ataxic gait*. See if the patient consistently staggers or turns to one side by asking them to march up and down on the spot with their eyes open and then shut. In Unterberger's test, the patient marches on the spot with the arms held out in front with the hands clasped; rotation is observed in a unilateral labyrinthine lesion. Get them to walk heel to toe and to walk round a chair, first one way and then the other. In a lesion of one cerebellar hemisphere they will consistently stagger to the side of the lesion (look for intention tremor and incoordination in the limbs, nystagmus and dysarthria). In midline cerebellar lesions the patient will stagger in any direction. The trunk may tilt when the patient is seated. Often, there is no other evidence of cerebellar disturbance such as intention tremor, nystagmus or dysarthria.

- Patients with involuntary movement disorders often have distinctive gaits:

  - The patient walks with the head twisted to one side (torticollis).
  - The head, trunk and limbs assume bizarre postures, often with associated abnormal movements (e.g. torsion dystonia).
  - Constant twitches in all parts of the body interrupt the normal smooth flow of movement, causing lurching and staggering. There may be facial grimacing and abnormal posturing of the limbs or trunk. These are features of the gait in Huntington's disease).
  - There are continuous writhing movements of the limbs during walking; one foot tends to invert, interfering with walking (e.g. 'dopa-induced dyskinesia' in a patient with Parkinson's disease).

- Patients who experience pain in the leg on bearing weight develop a very characteristic gait. You can see it for yourself by walking in front of a mirror with a pebble in your shoe. Each time you bear weight on the painful side, you hurry through the stride with the good leg to minimize the duration of the pain. The painful leg also buckles each time it bears weight in order to cushion the impact. This is called an *antalgic gait*. It is usually associated with arthritis of the hip, knee, ankle or foot joints.

Box 6.2 TIPS

- A shuffling gait with small steps and loss of arm swing is likely to be due to idiopathic Parkinson's disease if the base is normal. A shuffling gait but with a widened base is seen in normal-pressure hydrocephalus and the multi-lacunar state. The base is often also widened in the Parkinsonian disorder Progressive Supranuclear Gaze Palsy (Steele Richardson syndrome).[4]

- Romberg observed that patients with loss of proprioception due to tabes dorsalis toppled when asked to stand with their feet together and eyes closed. An increase in body sway following closure of the eyes is often accepted as a positive Romberg's sign. Unfortunately, this can occur when balance is impaired for any reason, and even in normal, anxious individuals. The term 'positive Rombergism' is, therefore, better reserved for patients who can stand unassisted, but would fall on closing the eyes if you did not prevent them. Do not attempt this test on a patient who is larger than you are without assistance.

- Most patients who have difficulty in walking will have evidence, when you come to examine them on the couch, of weakness, spasticity, rigidity, akinesia, sensory loss, or ataxia. If none of these is present, consider the possibility of a truncal ataxia due to a midline cerebellar lesion; alcoholism is the commonest cause of this. Another possibility is an apraxia of gait due to a frontal lobe lesion, though such a patient would be unlikely to be selected as a short case.

4. J Clifford Richardson, Canadian neurologist (1909–1886).

Facial palsy

7

Likely introduction: 'Examine the face' or 'Facial weakness'.

The facial muscles are supplied by the 7th cranial nerve, which arises from the facial nucleus in the pons (Fig. 7.1). The facial nerve is accompanied, for part of its course, by the chorda tympani, which innervates the taste receptors of the anterior two-thirds of the tongue. The muscles of the forehead are represented in the ipsilateral, as well as the contralateral, cerebral hemisphere (Fig. 7.2). Stroke is the commonest cause of an upper motor neurone facial palsy, and Bell's[1] palsy the commonest cause of a lower motor neurone palsy. Other causes of facial palsy are rare. The site of the lesion causing facial palsy is

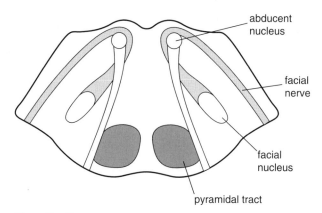

Figure 7.1 Transverse section of the pons.

1. *Sir Charles Bell, Scottish anatomist and surgeon (1774–1842).*

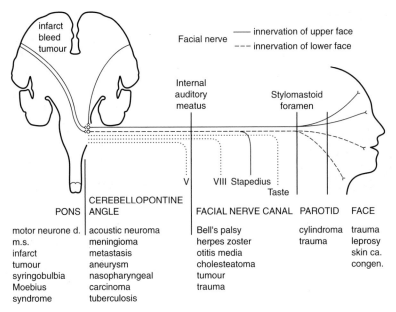

Figure 7.2 Schematic representation of the course and relations of the facial nerve.

PONS	CEREBELLOPONTINE ANGLE	FACIAL NERVE CANAL	PAROTID	FACE
motor neurone d.	acoustic neuroma	Bell's palsy	cylindroma	trauma
m.s.	meningioma	herpes zoster	trauma	leprosy
infarct	metastasis	otitis media		skin ca.
tumour	aneurysm	cholesteatoma		congen.
syringobulbia	nasopharyngeal	tumour		
Moebius	carcinoma	trauma		
syndrome	tuberculosis			

assessed by noting: (i) the pattern of facial weakness; and (ii) the presence of other signs.

Inspection

- Are there vesicles behind the ear, within the external meatus, or on the palate? (geniculate herpes, the Ramsay Hunt syndrome).[2]
- Is there evidence of a parotid mass or swelling (cylindroma, sarcoidosis)?
- When the patient blinks, does the corner of the mouth twitch? When the patient smiles, does the eye close more on the affected side? These are features of synkinesis ('cross-talk' between axons within the facial nerve) and signify that the lesion is long-standing. Pouting is better than smiling for revealing eye closure due to synkinesis.
- Is the naso-labial fold (Fig. 7.3) lost (confirming weakness of the facial muscles) or deepened (signifying a long-standing weakness and associated with synkinesis)?

2. *James Ramsay Hunt, American neurologist (1872–1937).*

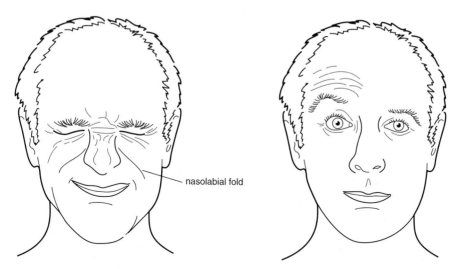

Figure 7.3 Raising the eyebrows: selective lesion of the temporal branch of the facial nerve.

- Look for scars on the face (previous surgery for skin cancers) and over the occiput (previous surgery for acoustic neuroma).

Distribution of weakness

Ask the patient to:

- Raise the eyebrows. Some patients have difficulty doing this voluntarily, but will do it involuntarily when asked to look up at the ceiling.
- Screw the eyes up tightly. Observe whether the eyelashes are buried.
- Show me your teeth.
- Blow the cheeks out. Air will escape from the mouth if there is weakness of orbicularis oris, and the cheek will blow out more on the side where there is weakness of buccinator.
- Turn your mouth down. This will also cause platysma to contract in many patients.

There are four main patterns of weakness:

- Weakness of all the muscles on one side of the face except frontalis and orbicularis oculi. The patient has an upper motor neurone lesion. This is most commonly due to a stroke involving the contralateral cerebral hemisphere and the facial weakness is but one part of a hemiparesis (detectable with your screening tests). Patients with this type of facial weakness often elevate the angle of the mouth involuntarily when smiling, but cannot do so on command.

- Weakness of all the muscles on one side of the face. The patient has a lower motor neurone lesion, usually due to Bell's palsy. In Bell's palsy, there is often loss of taste and hyperacusis but no other signs. If it is due to a lesion of the facial nucleus, the patient may also have a CN VI nerve palsy or gaze palsy on the same side (see Fig. 7.2). If it is due to tumour – for example, acoustic neuroma or infection within the facial nerve canal – there may also be deafness or loss of taste.
- Bilateral facial weakness. When this occurs acutely, it is usually due to Guillain–Barré syndrome, and there may be associated generalized weakness and areflexia (Box 7.1). Other causes of bilateral facial weakness or loss of facial movement include:

Box 7.1 Management issues in acute peripheral neuropathy.

Investigations

- Nerve conduction studies to determine if it is axonal or demyelinating. *N.B.* Conduction may be normal distally. Look for conduction block proximally
- Cerebrospinal fluid (CSF) protein elevated in Guillain–Barré syndrome
- Antibodies: GQ1b GM1
- Infections: hepatitis C, HIV, *Campylobacter*

Treatment

- Protect the airway, avoid aspiration, ventilation
- Supportive: chest physiotherapy, 'thromboembolism prevention stockings'
- Plasma exchange, immunoglobulin
- Manage postural hypotension

- Sarcoidosis (with parotid swelling and fever).
- Myopathies such as facio-scapulo-humeral dystrophy, oculopharyngeal dystrophy or mitochondrial myopathy.
- Dystrophia myotonica (with ptosis, wasting of the masseters and sternomastoids, cataracts, frontal balding and inability to release the hand grip).
- Myasthenia gravis (with ptosis and diplopia which worsen with sustained contraction and rapidly improve with rest. The pupils are spared. There may also be proximal weakness of the limbs).
- Parkinson's disease. The 'frozen features' of the patient with Parkinson's disease are not due to weakness, but to akinesia. These patients are able to bury their eyelashes and blow their cheeks out.
- Bilateral upper motor neurone facial weakness occurs in multilacunar states (pseudobulbar palsy) and motor neurone disease. There is usually a brisk jaw jerk. While these patients have difficulty voluntarily contracting the facial muscles, their expressions may change in an exaggerated manner, and they may laugh or cry inappropriately.

- Weakness confined to one or two facial muscles on the same side (rare). In Fig. 7.3, for example, weakness is confined to frontalis. This is never seen acutely in Bell's palsy; it may occur following incomplete recovery from a Bell's palsy and is then associated with synkinesis. Such a selective weakness is usually due to a lesion of the facial nerve after it has divided into its terminal branches in the parotid gland. Causes include: facial trauma, parotid tumour, leprosy, and perineural spread from a skin cancer.

Sensation on the face

Test touch and pin prick sensation on the forehead, cheek and chin on both sides of the face. Check corneal sensation. Several types of finding are worth considering:

- It is normal in Bell's palsy. Absence of the corneal reflex in Bell's palsy is due to interruption of the efferent limb of the reflex arc; the other eye blinks briskly when the cornea on the paralysed side is touched.

- In acoustic neuroma there is usually loss of corneal sensation, and neither eye blinks when the cornea on the affected side is touched. Facial sensation is otherwise normal. Facial weakness is slight and there is deafness.
- Facial numbness, as part of a hemianaesthesia, is seen with strokes.
- Loss of sensation on the face, in the distribution of terminal branches of the trigeminal nerve, is a feature of perineural spread from skin cancers.
- Loss of sensation in the coolest parts of the face (nose and ears) is characteristic of leprosy (rare).
- Dissociated sensory loss on the face is seen in brainstem lesions such as syringobulbia or glioma. Pain sensation is lost, and touch sensation is preserved. The pattern of sensory loss with central lesions follows an 'onion-peel' pattern (Fig. 7.4), unlike sensory loss from peripheral lesions of the trigeminal nerve (Fig. 7.5).

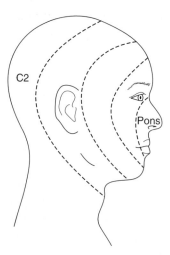

Figure 7.4 'Onion-peel' distribution of sensory loss associated with central lesions of the trigeminal nerve.

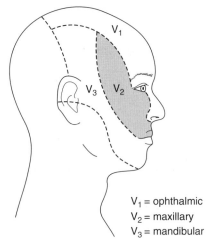

V_1 = ophthalmic
V_2 = maxillary
V_3 = mandibular

Figure 7.5 Distribution of sensory loss associated with peripheral lesions of the trigeminal nerve.

Taste

The testing of taste is time-consuming, and you will not be expected to do this in a short case. You should mention it, however, when discussing the case with the examiners. Taste sensation is normal in upper motor neurone facial weakness and in lesions of the facial nerve after it has left the facial canal. It is often lost in Bell's palsy and other lesions within the facial canal.

Other important signs to look for

- Ptosis. The combination of weakness of orbicularis oculi and ptosis, with normal pupillary function, usually signifies that the problem involves muscle or neuromuscular function (see above).
- Bilateral ophthalmoplegia. This again usually signifies muscle disease or myasthenia gravis, the pupils being spared. Another cause of facial weakness and ophthalmoplegia is the Miller Fisher variant of Guillain–Barré syndrome.
- Hearing. The combination of deafness and facial palsy is seen in lesions of the cerebello-pontine angle (e.g. acoustic neuroma) or of the facial canal (see Fig. 7.2). Hyperacusis often occurs in Bell's palsy due to paralysis of the nerve to stapedius.
- Facial swelling (rare) occurs in the Melkersson–Rosenthal syndrome. Here, the facial palsy is often recurrent. Facial swelling also occurs in parotid tumours and parotitis due to sarcoid.

Box 7.2 TIPS

- In an acute 'upper motor neurone' facial weakness, frontalis is often weak for a few days. At this time it may be indistinguishable from a 'lower motor neurone' weakness.
- The elevators of the eyelids are not supplied by the facial nerve. Ptosis is not, therefore, a feature of a facial nerve lesion. A confusing sign is narrowing of the palpebral fissure due to over-activity of the orbicularis oculi muscle. This is seen in long-standing Bell's palsy and is associated with deepening of the naso-labial fold and a dimple in the chin.
- Facial palsy, occurring immediately after a fracture of the petrous part of the temporal bone, usually does not improve, as the nerve is severed. When it occurs several days after the head injury, recovery is the rule.

- In multiple sclerosis, facial palsy – unlike weakness in other muscle groups – is often 'lower motor neurone' in type. This may be due to demyelination of the nerve during its relatively long course within the pons, after leaving the facial nucleus (see Fig. 7.1).

- Many patients with Bell's palsy complain of a slight alteration of sensation on the affected side. This can be safely ignored, provided that the patient can feel the lightest touch, tell one end of the pin from the other, and has a normal consensual blink reflex.

- The affected eye sometimes brims with tears. This is due to separation of the punctum of the lacrimal duct from the conjunctival surface. It is not due to excessive production of tears. To the contrary, lachrymation is often reduced in Bell's palsy due to involvement of parasympathetic nerves.

- Bilateral facial weakness is easy to miss, as the patient's features are symmetrical. It should be suspected when, during the course of giving you the history, the patient is unblinking, expressionless, and smiles 'horizontally' – that is, they fail to elevate the angles of the mouth. Speech is often impaired – particularly labial sounds like 'puh' – and the patient cannot form a seal with the lips when asked to blow the cheeks out. In severe cases the eyes are seen to roll up as the patient blinks (Bell's phenomenon).

- Bell's phenomenon is useful for determining whether a patient is really trying to screw the eyes up. Unless there is paralysis of the extra-ocular muscles, the eyes roll up when the orbicularis oculi muscles contract forcefully.

- Beware the child with an acute Bell's palsy where there is a recognized association with hypertension.

- Finally, do not overdiagnose facial palsy. Many patients have a lopsided smile and they will soon tell you that this has always been the case, if you ask them. An old photograph is helpful.

Ptosis

Likely introduction: 'Drooping of the eyelid(s)' or 'Examine the face'.

Drooping of the eyelids is common in the elderly, and results from dehiscence of the levator aponeurosis. In the context of a neurology short case it usually results from weakness of the levator palpebrae superioris muscle. This is innervated by the oculomotor (IIIrd) nerve. The under-surface of the levator muscles is connected to the tarsus by smooth muscle fibres, Muller's muscle, which is innervated by cervical sympathetic nerves. Ptosis results from damage to these nerves or to disorders of muscle or neuromuscular junction.

Inspection

Give yourself a moment to take in the overall appearance of the patient. There are some characteristic presentations:

- One eye closed, the other normal (oculomotor palsy or myasthenia gravis).
- Ptosis on one side with the pupil larger on the same side (oculomotor palsy; Fig. 8.1).
- Partial ptosis on one side with the pupil smaller on the same side (Horner's syndrome; Fig. 8.1).
- Bilateral ptosis (myopathy such as dystrophia myotonica [drooping mouth, thin neck and frontal balding] or Kearns–Sayre syndrome; or myasthenia gravis).
- Proptosis and ptosis in one eye (orbital tumour or vascular anomaly). Listen for a bruit over the eye.

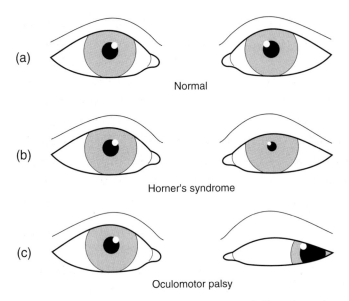

Figure 8.1 The eyes in the primary position: normal, Horner's syndrome, oculomotor nerve palsy.

Distribution of weakness

In the first place, you need to:

- test visual acuity;
- examine the lens and fundi;
- test pupillary response to light and accommodation;
- test visual fields;
- test eye movements; and
- examine for weakness of the facial muscles (especially orbicularis oculi).

What you find will then lead you to other aspects of the examination. Certain patterns of weakness are characteristic:

- Unilateral ptosis:

  - With the patient attempting to look straight ahead, the eye is 'down and out' (see Fig. 8.1c). There is weakness of adduction and vertical eye movements; the pupil is fixed and dilated. The patient has an *oculomotor (IIIrd) nerve palsy* (see Chapter 9).

- As for the previous case, but with pupillary sparing. Consider small-vessel disease due to diabetes mellitus and/or hypertension as a cause.
- With the pupil smaller on the same side but normally reactive to light, eye movements are full (see Fig. 8.1b). The patient has a *Horner's syndrome*. If you look carefully, you may note that the lower lid is elevated on the affected side. Brush the back of your hand across the forehead. The skin may feel moist and sticky on the normal side, but smooth on the anhidrotic side. Horner's syndrome is a good lateralizing but a poor localizing sign as the cervical sympathetic fibres run such a tortuous course. The following associated signs should be particularly looked for:

  - Loss of the corneal reflex in the same eye (orbital or retro-orbital lesion);
  - Weakness and loss of reflexes in the ipsilateral arm (avulsion injury to the brachial plexus; Pancoast[1] tumour of the lung apex);
  - Ipsilateral loss of facial pain and temperature sensation and con-tralateral loss of pain and temperature sensation in the trunk and limbs (brainstem lesion).

- With (or without) weakness of extra-ocular muscles and orbicularis oculi consider *myasthenia gravis* (Box 8.1). Ask the patient to look up at the ceiling for about 2 minutes. The ptosis may worsen. After a brief rest, the eyelid will resume its original position. Look for evidence of weakness and fatigability in the limbs. Fatigability is most conveniently tested in the deltoid muscles. Sit the patient in a chair and ask them to abduct the arms at the shoulder, flex the elbows and to resist your attempts to press their arms down. It is easier for you to sustain this by pressing repetitively (about once per second) rather than continuously. Within a minute or so it becomes progressively easier to press the arms down if the patient has myasthenia gravis. Again, after a brief rest the muscle strength returns. Triceps is often weak in myasthenia gravis.

- Bilateral ptosis

- With normal pupils. This usually signifies a disorder of muscle or neuro-muscular junction. If there is weakness of the extra-ocular muscles and of orbicularis oculi, the following should be considered:

1. *Henry Khunrath Pancoast, American radiologist and radiotherapist (1875–1939).*

Box 8.1 Management issues in myasthenia gravis.

Investigations

- Respiratory function tests
- Modified barium swallow
- Repetitive stimulation studies
- Single-fibre electromyography (EMG) looking for jitter
- Anti-acetylcholine receptor antibodies (Anti-MuSK antibodies if negative)
- Edrophonium (Tensilon) test
- Computed tomography of the chest to exclude thymoma

Treatment

- Acutely might include: plasma exchange, gamma globulin, steroids, anticholinesterase drugs (pyridistigmine)
- Supportive: airway protection, ventilation
- Thymectomy

- Senile ptosis (see Tips).
- Ocular myopathy. In Kearns–Sayre syndrome, there is complete or partial ophthalmoplegia with ptosis which may be unilateral or asymmetrical and the pupils are normal. In other myopathies there may be generalized weakness. Ask for the ECG to see if there is a conduction defect.

- Myasthenia gravis (see above).
- Dystrophia myotonica. Supporting evidence will include frontal balding, cataracts, wasting of the masseters, sternomastoids and distal limb muscles. Again, ask for the ECG to see if there is a conduction defect. Test for myotonia (see section on wasting of the hand).

- With unreactive dilated pupils. This uncommon finding is likely to be due to an abnormality of the oculomotor nerves (such as Miller Fisher syndrome) or their central connections in the midbrain.

Box 8.2 TIPS

- Complete ptosis, where the pupil is covered by the lid, is unlikely to be due to Horner's syndrome.
- Pupillary inequality due to an oculomotor palsy is most obvious in a well-lit room; due to Horner's syndrome, is most obvious in a dimly lit room.
- Ptosis associated with weakness of orbicularis oculi is likely to be due to myasthenia gravis or to an ocular myopathy.
- Always consider myasthenia gravis when the pattern of weakness of eye movements cannot be readily fitted into a IIIrd, IVth or VIth cranial nerve palsy (and even when it can).
- In unilateral Horner's syndrome which has been present from birth, the iris of the affected eye may remain blue when the other becomes brown (heterochromia).
- In dysthyroid eye disease, ophthalmoplegia is usually associated with lid retraction, not ptosis.
- A common cause of bilateral ptosis (though probably not one that would appear in a short case) is 'mechanical' ptosis where the levator palpebrae muscle dehisces from the tarsal plate. This condition is seen in elderly patients, and is often called 'senile ptosis'. There are no associated neurological signs.
- In ptosis associated with a complete IIIrd nerve palsy there is often mild proptosis when the patient is examined sitting up. This is due to loss of tone in the extra-ocular muscles; it disappears when the patient lies down.

Abnormalities of vision or eye movement

9

Inspection

Testing vision

The remainder of the examination

Likely introduction: 'Poor vision', 'Double vision', or 'Examine the eyes'.

To see properly you need to have normal eyes, eye movements and central visual connections. Your approach to the examination thus involves determining which of these three components has failed. The range of possibilities with this introduction is wide and includes: blindness in one eye, bitemporal hemianopia, homonymous hemianopia and IIIrd, IVth or VIth nerve palsies. Patients with pupillary abnormalities and nystagmus will also be considered in this chapter. Many candidates experience difficulty in testing the eyes, and some time will be spent in describing techniques which are useful.

Inspection

Step back and look at the patient as a whole. Certain features may be very revealing:

- Acromegaly or the smooth, soft, 'feminine' cheeks (in a man) signifying hypopituitarism. In such patients you will be looking carefully for a bitemporal hemianopia.
- A patient with an obvious hemiparesis may also have a homonymous hemianopia, though this is only one of many associations.
- Loss of facial expression and ptosis raise the possibility of disorders of muscle or the neuromuscular junction (myopathy, myasthenia gravis, dystrophia myotonica).

- Look carefully at the eyes for nystagmus, inequality of the pupils, proptosis, cataracts and evidence of trauma.

Testing vision

Test the following in every patient:

- **Acuity.** In the context of a short case it is probably not necessary to check near and far vision. Carry a card with letters of different sizes which you give the patient to hold at a comfortable reading distance. See what the patient can read (with reading glasses if they are normally used). Ask them if they wear reading glasses and to use them if they do. The aim of this part of the exercise is to make sure that the patient is not blind or near-blind in one or both eyes. Subtle abnormalities of visual acuity are not a concern.
- **Fundoscopy.** Maximize your chances of seeing something other than the reflection of the light from your ophthalmoscope by dimming the lights in the room, using a narrow beam and using, initially, a low light strength. Get as much practice as you can in using the instrument. It is very obvious in an examination situation if you are unfamiliar with the technique. The main abnormalities you are likely to encounter are papilloedema, optic atrophy, cataracts or gross retinal changes such as diabetic retinopathy, hypertensive retinopathy, haemorrhages and retinitis pigmentosa. If you are unable to visualize the retina, consider the possibility of cataracts or opacities in the cornea or vitreous humour.
- **Fields.** Visual field testing is often done badly and obvious abnormalities missed. The following approach may help:
  - *Peripheral field testing.* Sit in front of the patient, as shown in Fig. 9.1. The patient has both eyes open. Hold both of your hands in the upper fields and ask the patient to look at your eyes and to point to where your fingers are moving. Explain that sometimes you will move your fingers on both sides together. Move your fingers on one side, then the other, then both together. Repeat the procedure in the lower fields. This technique is good for detecting homonymous hemianopia and visual neglect. In the latter,

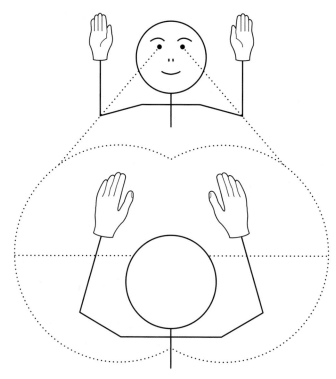

Figure 9.1 Testing the quadrants of the peripheral visual field.

the patient will miss the movements in the left visual field only when there are simultaneous movements in the right field. It is not good at detecting a blind eye for the field of a single eye is wide.

- *Central field testing* (Fig. 9.2). Cup your hand over your left eye and ask the patient to do the same with their right eye (warn the patient not to press on the eye or it will be untestable for the next few minutes). Ask the patient to look at your eye. Place a red pin head in each of the four quadrants of the visual field, close to its centre. Ask the patient whether they can see the pin and whether the colour is the same in each quadrant. Don't stray far from the centre of the field; you will see yourself that the colour fades the further out you go. This is a sensitive test for optic nerve and chiasmal lesions; the patient will not see the pin on the affected side, or it will look grey. You can also assess the size of the blind spot in someone with papilloedema.

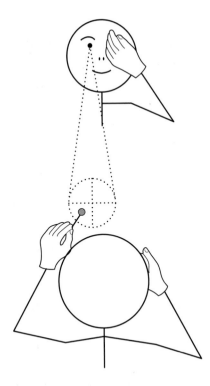

Figure 9.2 Testing the quadrants of the central visual field with a red pin.

- **Pupillary responses.** See if the pupils are equal. Ask the patient to fixate on the wall opposite and test the direct and consensual light reflexes. An absent light reflex is a key sign and should be checked carefully. A common cause of failure to induce a light reflex on the wards is a flat torch battery. Sometimes it is difficult to see the response in a brightly lit room because the pupils are so constricted. If in doubt, dim the lights. Use the swinging torch test to detect a relative afferent pupillary defect (the Marcus Gunn[1] response): shine the light in one eye and then quickly flick it across to the other eye, wait a second or two, then flick it back. Each time the light hits the eye with impaired vision, the pupil dilates. Test the near reflex.

- **Eye movements.** Observe the position of the eyes and look for evidence of strabismus (squint) or nystagmus in the primary position (looking straight ahead). Here are some techniques which may prove useful:

  - **Testing eye movements**

    - *Pursuit gaze testing.* Ask the patient to follow your finger as you trace a large figure 'H'; this causes the eyes to move horizontally and then verti-

---

1. *Robert Marcus Gunn, Scottish ophthalmologist (1850–1909).*

cally in the abducted and adducted positions. Check the range of movement achieved by each eye and whether the movements are smooth as
they follow your finger; in cerebellar disorders they are often jerky.

- *Voluntary gaze testing.* First, ask the patient to look to the left, then to
  the right, then up, then down. This will give you an idea of the range
  of eye movements. Note whether the patient blinks to initiate gaze or
  moves their head rather than their eyes. With practice, you may
  notice whether the saccades are slow. (The saccades are eye movements generated in a voluntary gaze, and are so rapid that you cannot
  see them, only their start and finish.) These disorders of voluntary
  gaze are characteristic of certain diseases such as Progressive
  Supranuclear Gaze Palsy (PSP), Huntington's disease[2] and the rare
  Spinocerebellar Ataxia (SCA II & VII) (Box 9.1). Now, hold the
  thumb of your left hand and the index finger of your right hand
  about 50 cm apart in front of the patient. Ask the patient to look at
  your thumb when it moves and then your finger (again, when it
  moves). See if their eyes can go from one digit to the other in one
  clean sweep (saccade). The hallmark of motor dysfunction in
  Parkinson's disease is loss of amplitude of voluntary movements. In
  the eyes, this is reflected as hypometric saccades, with the eyes

---

Box 9.1 Management issues in cerebellar syndromes.

Investigations

- Computed tomography (CT)/MRI to exclude infarct/tumour
- Thyroid function tests
- Chest X-ray (paraneoplastic)
- Genetic tests for spinocerebellar ataxia (SCA)
- Anti-neuronal antibodies (paraneoplastic syndrome), anti-
  endomysial antibodies (coeliac disease)

Treatment

- Symptomatic
- Genetic counselling

---

2. *George Sumner Huntington, American neurologist (1851–1916).*

moving from thumb to finger in a series of bunny-hops rather than in one leap. In cerebellar disorders, the eyes may overshoot the target and then return (ocular dysmetria). In PSP, the patient may not be able to look down voluntarily and yet will achieve a full vertical excursion if the examiner passively flexes and extends the head as the patient fixates on a target (the doll's head eye movement or oculo-cephalic manoeuvre induced by the vestibulo-ocular reflex).

- **The cover test**

  - *Objective confirmation of diplopia.* Failure of one or both eyes to move in a certain direction may be obvious. Often it is not, though the patient may complain of seeing double. You may confirm that the eyes are not aligned using the cover test. Ask the patient to fixate on your pin with both eyes open. Move the pin around until you find the position where the patient says that they are seeing double. Now cover each eye in turn. The eye that is fixating will not move when the other is covered. The other eye will move when the fixating eye is covered.
  - The traditional method of determining which muscle is weak is to cover each eye in turn and to ask the patient which of the two images has disappeared. The outer image comes from the eye which has not moved fully. Unfortunately, patients often have difficulty with this test and report that it is the outer image which has gone when either eye is covered. It is more useful to determine from the patient whether the two images are separated in the vertical (e.g. IIIrd and IVth nerve palsies) or horizontal (e.g. VIth nerve palsy) planes.

The remainder of the examination

You now have enough information to proceed with the remainder of the examination. What you do next will depend upon what you have found:

- **Abnormality of vision.** Here, you have found impairment of the visual fields or acuity. This might consist of:

  - **Impairment of acuity in one eye** (Fig. 9.3a). Cover the other eye and see if the patient can perceive hand movements or the light of your torch.

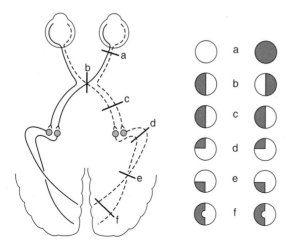

Figure 9.3 Examples of visual field losses and their associated lesions.

The pupils are equal, but the affected eye has no response to light or has a relative afferent pupillary defect. The problem lies in the anterior visual system: the eye itself (e.g. central retinal artery occlusion, retinitis pigmentosa) or the optic nerve. If there is swelling of the optic disc, consider conditions such as optic neuritis or ischaemic optic neuropathy (see Tips). If there is optic atrophy, a number of possibilities exist: sub-frontal meningioma (test smell); pituitary tumour; carotid aneurysm; anterior ischaemic optic neuropathy (feel the superficial temporal pulses and ask what the ESR is as temporal arteritis can cause this); multiple sclerosis; trauma; syphilis.

- **Bitemporal hemianopia** (Fig. 9.3b). This signifies a lesion of the optic chiasm, most commonly due to a pituitary tumour. You may have already observed the changes of hypopituitarism or acromegaly. Ask if the patient has galactorrhoea (prolactinoma).
- **Homonymous hemianopia** (Fig. 9.3c and f). This signifies a lesion behind the optic chiasm – that is, involving the optic tract, radiation or visual cortex. In a left homonymous hemianopia, look for evidence of non-dominant parietal lobe function. Get the patient to draw a clock, put a cross in the middle of a line, and copy a cube. Test for sensory neglect. Use your screening tests to detect a hemiparesis. In a right homonymous hemianopia look for evidence of aphasia and again for hemiparesis. Test reading. The commonest causes of homonymous hemianopia with these signs are stroke and tumour.

- **Upper homonymous quadrantanopia** (see Fig. 9.3d). This signifies a temporal lobe lesion; a **lower homonymous quadrantanopia** signifies a parietal lobe lesion (Fig. 9.3e).

- **Abnormality of eye movements.** This is likely to be one of two types:

  - **Weak eye muscles**

Here, there is weakness of the ocular muscles of one or both eyes:

  - The patient fails to abduct one eye (Fig. 9.4). There are no other ocular findings. The patient has weakness of the lateral rectus muscle, most commonly due to an abducens (VIth) nerve palsy. The abducens nucleus is in the pons: check facial sensation and use the screening tests, looking for a contralateral hemiparesis (see Fig. 7.1). Causes of abducens palsy include microvascular occlusion of the vasa nervorum of the VIth nerve due to hypertension or diabetes, raised intracranial pressure, cavernous sinus lesions and nasopharyngeal carcinoma. Often, no cause is found.

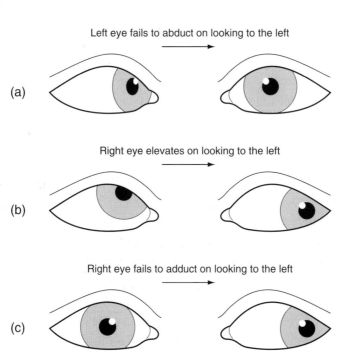

Left eye fails to abduct on looking to the left

(a)

Right eye elevates on looking to the left

(b)

Right eye fails to adduct on looking to the left

(c)

Figure 9.4 (a) Left abducens nerve palsy; (b) right trochlear nerve palsy; (c) right internuclear ophthalmoplegia.

– In the primary position, one eye assumes an abducted and depressed position (Fig. 8.1c). There is weakness of adduction, elevation and depression of the eye, and ptosis. The pupil is fixed and dilated. The patient has an oculomotor (IIIrd) nerve palsy. When this occurs acutely and there is a pain in the eye, it is a matter of some urgency to exclude a posterior communicating aneurysm (with a CT angiogram, MRA or spiral angiogram). Clipping the aneurysm before it has ruptured carries a much lower mortality than after. Chronic meningitis (e.g. tuberculosis), raised intracranial pressure or cavernous sinus lesions (check trigeminal nerve function) may also cause IIIrd nerve palsies. The pupil is characteristically spared in a IIIrd nerve palsy associated with diabetes mellitus or hypertension.

– On looking to the left, the right eye rides up (Fig. 9.4b). The head is tilted to the left. The patient has weakness of the right superior oblique muscle, usually due to a trochlear (IVth) nerve palsy. Attempts to demonstrate failure of the eye to depress in the adducted position are usually unrewarding. Often, it follows head injury, but diabetes is another cause.

– On lateral gaze, one eye fails to adduct (or adducts slowly) and the abducting eye overshoots and then corrects (Fig. 9.4c) or shows nystagmus. The affected eye may adduct fully on convergence testing. The patient has a unilateral internuclear ophthalmoplegia (INO). This signifies a lesion of the medial longitudinal fasciculus (Fig. 9.5). Unilateral INO is often due to stroke, and bilateral INO to multiple sclerosis.

– Mild limitation of upward gaze is a common finding in otherwise normal elderly patients and in Parkinson's disease.

– Both eyes fail to look to one side (conjugate gaze palsy). Loss of voluntary lateral gaze usually signifies a lesion of the contralateral frontal lobe or the ipsilateral pons (see Fig. 9.5).

– On attempted upward gaze, the eyes develop a rapid flickering motion towards each other and retract rhythmically. This is convergence–retraction nystagmus, and is a feature of Parinaud's syndrome.[3] The pupils may also become unreactive to light but not to accommodation. The usual underlying cause is compression of the midbrain by a pinealoma. Other causes include hydrocephalus and stroke.

3. Henri Parinaud, French neuro-ophthalmologist (1844–1905).

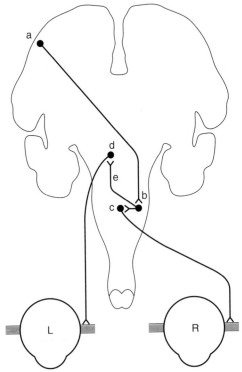

Figure 9.5 Pathway for lateral gaze. a, frontal lobe eye field; b, pontine lateral gaze centre; c, abducens nucleus; d, medial rectus nucleus of the oculomotor nerve; e, medial longitudinal faciculus.

   – Loss of downward gaze. In an elderly patient this is likely to be due to progressive supranuclear palsy (PSP; Steele Richardson syndrome), a type of parkinsonism. There is also loss of upward gaze. While the patient cannot look up or down voluntarily or with pursuit, reflex movement is preserved, showing that the lesion is above the nucleus of the oculomotor and trochlear nerves (i.e. it is 'supranuclear'). Ask the patient to look at a point on the wall opposite. Now, tilt the head back (this may be difficult as there is often marked neck rigidity in PSP, in itself a helpful sign). The eyes will depress.

● **Nystagmus.** This refers to involuntary rhythmical movements of the eyes. In most cases each movement has a fast and a slow phase ('jerk' nystagmus). Note whether the nystagmus is present in the primary position (looking straight ahead), on horizontal gaze, or on vertical gaze. Does it beat in a horizontal (left or right) or vertical plane (up or down)? By convention, the direction of nystagmus is defined by the direction of the fast phase. Vestibular nystagmus can be either 'peripheral' (labyrinth) or 'central' (vestibular nucleus/cerebellum), and is often induced by head movement. Patients with peripheral nystagmus may have deafness and tinnitus, but usually no other signs. Patients with nystagmus of brainstem origin often have a plethora of neurological signs making them ideal for short cases! Gaze-evoked nystagmus is typically due to brainstem or cerebellar lesions. Several examples of nystagmus are worthy of mention.

- A few beats of horizontal nystagmus, only present at the extremes of lateral gaze. Unsustained nystagmus of this type is physiological. Avoid moving the eyes beyond the range of comfortable binocular vision.
- Fine horizontal nystagmus with the fast component to one or other side, only present on deviation of the eyes to that side. This could be due to a peripheral or central lesion. Peripheral vestibular nystagmus beats away from the side of the lesion, whatever the direction of the gaze. Cerebellar nystagmus is gaze-evoked and typically beats to the side of the lesion if unilateral, but may also beat in whichever direction the patient looks. Central vestibular nystagmus, if purely horizontal, will usually beat away from the side of the lesion whichever way the patient looks. In such a patient you should:
    - Test hearing. Whisper a number on one side while masking the other ear by rubbing the tragus against the external meatus. Hearing might be impaired in a peripheral lesion as in Menières disease. It might also be impaired in a cerebellopontine angle tumour. If hearing is impaired, you would be expected to do Rinné and Weber tests though, in the noisy environment of a ward or clinic, these are rarely helpful.
    - Test facial and corneal sensation and look for facial weakness (cerebellopontine angle tumour or pontine lesion).
    - Look for cerebellar signs: dysarthria, intention tremor, ataxic gait.
    - Perform screening tests for a hemiparesis.
- Sustained horizontal nystagmus on lateral gaze in both directions. This is seen in patients who are intoxicated with drugs such as phenytoin, benzodiazepines and barbiturates. They may also have dysarthria and

limb ataxia. It may also result from the lesions of the cerebellum and brainstem mentioned.

- Vertical nystagmus. This usually signifies a central lesion. It can be caused by the same drugs as horizontal nystagmus. There are two main types of vertical nystagmus:
    - Upbeat nystagmus, where the fast phase is upwards. Causes include multiple sclerosis, stroke, tumour and Wernicke's[4] encephalopathy. It is also seen in bilateral internuclear ophthalmoplegia.
    - Downbeat nystagmus, where the fast phase is downwards, is less common, and is particularly associated with lesions of the cervicomedullary junction such as the Arnold–Chiari[5] malformation.
    - Nystagmus confined to one eye ('ataxic' nystagmus) is seen in an internuclear ophthalmoplegia (see above).
    - Convergence–retraction nystagmus is seen in lesions of the tectal plate of the midbrain (see above).
    - In pendular nystagmus there are no clearly recognizable fast and slow phases; the movements are sinusoidal. It is often long-standing and associated with failure of visual fixation or blindness. A common cause is multiple sclerosis.

- **Pupillary abnormality**. This is likely to be one of the following:

- One pupil is smaller than the other. Both react briskly to light and accommodation. There is ptosis on the side of the small pupil. The patient has Horner's syndrome (see Fig 8.1b).
- One pupil is smaller than the other. The larger pupil is unreactive to light or accommodation. There is ptosis and limitation of eye movements on the side with the larger pupil. The patient has a IIIrd nerve palsy (see Fig 8.1c).
- One or both pupils are large, react poorly to light, but do constrict to a near stimulus. There is no ptosis; eye movements are full. This is likely to an Adie[6] ('tonic') pupil; check for areflexia. Other possibilities include traumatic iridoplegia and the result of previous application of mydriatic eye drops.

---

4. *Karl Wernicke, German neuropsychiatrist (1848–1905).*
5. *Julius Arnold, German physician (1835–1915); Hans Chiari, Austrian pathologist (1851–1916).*
6. *William John Adie, Queen Square neurologist (1887–1935).*

- Both pupils are small, irregular, and unreactive to light. The response to accommodation is preserved. There is no ptosis. Eye movements are full. The patient may have Argyll Robertson[7] (A-R) pupils. A-R pupils are now rare and associated with diabetic autonomic neuropathy rather than neurosyphilis; more common is the long-standing Adie pupil which eventually becomes small. Like the A-R pupil, the response to accommodation is often brisk and, whilst the pupil does constrict to light, this may take so long as to be missed. The pupils of patients with glaucoma treated with pilocarpine eye drops are very small, and in these it may be difficult to see any response to light or accommodation.

Box 9.2 TIPS

- Optic nerve disease does not cause inequality of the pupils for the direct and consensual light reflexes are of equal strength. Thus, if the right optic nerve were transected, the size of the right pupil would remain the same as that of the left, by the action of the consensual reflex.
- The finding of an afferent pupillary defect usually indicates a lesion of the optic nerve, and is less common in retinal lesions.
- Optic disc swelling may be due to optic neuritis or raised intracranial pressure. In optic neuritis there is a central scotoma, impairment of colour vision (especially to red) and visual acuity is impaired; in raised intracranial pressure the blind spots are enlarged and the visual acuity is usually normal in the early stages.
- Myasthenia gravis may mimic a IIIrd, IVth or VIth cranial nerve palsy, and even an internuclear ophthalmoplegia. The pupil is spared and there is often weakness of orbicularis oculi. The signs are usually bilateral and there is ptosis. Fatigability is the key sign.
- Dysthyroid eye disease should always be considered if the abnormality of eye movement does not readily conform to a IIIrd, IVth or VIth cranial nerve palsy. Associated features include proptosis, lid lag, lid retraction and conjunctival injection.
- You will miss the important sign of visual neglect, usually signifying a non-dominant parietal lesion, unless you routinely test the patient with simultaneous stimuli in each half field.

7. DMCL Argyll Robertson, Scottish ophthalmologist (1837–1909).

- The obliques elevate and depress the eyes in the adducted position, the recti in the abducted position.
- Abnormalities of conjugate horizontal gaze are seen in lesions of the pons, frontal or occipital lobes. Conjugate vertical gaze is impaired in lesions of the midbrain.
- Nystagmus is likely to be of central origin if it is vertical or involves only one eye.
- Nystagmus, dysarthria and tremor are some of the acute effects of alcohol. Often the only cerebellar sign in a chronic alcoholic is unsteadiness of gait.
- In a young woman, who looks well and has no ocular signs apart from a dilated, slowly reactive pupil, consider the Holmes–Adie syndrome.[8] Often the pupil is oval. Both pupils may be involved. Check the tendon reflexes. In elderly patients with this syndrome, the pupils may become small.

8. Sir Gordon Holmes, Queen Square neurologist whose system of neurological examination forms the basis of what we all do to this day (1876–1965).

Tremor

10

Inspection
Examination of tremor
Other aspects

Likely introduction: 'Tremor of the hands' or 'Examine the upper limbs'.

Tremor is a rhythmical involuntary movement of any part of the body, but most commonly of the hands. It is convenient to divide tremors into three main categories: resting; postural; and intention. The commonest cause is physiological tremor, which you might have when you do the neurology short case. The patient is more likely to have Essential tremor or Parkinson's disease.

Inspection

Step back and look at the patient as a whole. You should have two questions in your mind:

- Which parts of the body are shaking? Look particularly at the lips, tongue, chin, head and limbs. You will need to comment on the distribution to the examiners.
- Are there any signs of Parkinson's disease? These might include: flexed posture, expressionless face, dribbling and poverty of movement (Box 10.1).

Examination of tremor

The next step is to define the characteristics of the tremor. This is done on the basis of two criteria:

Box 10.1 Management issues in Parkinson's disease.

Investigations

- Usually none
- MRI if it is suspected that the Parkinson's disease is not idiopathic
  - multi-lacunar state
  - multiple system atrophy: putamenal atrophy

Treatment

- Levodopa with decarboxylase inhibitor (DCI) catechol-ortho-methyltransferase (COMT) inhibitor
- Other drugs (agonists, selegiline, anticholinergics, amantadine)
- Surgery

- The circumstances in which it is maximal.
- Whether it is coarse (high amplitude, low frequency) or fine (low amplitude, high frequency).

Observe the tremor in the hands:

- with the patient sitting with their hands resting on their lap. A tremor that is maximal in this posture is called a **'resting tremor'** and is characteristic of Parkinson's disease. It is usually coarse and more marked in one hand than in the other. It pauses during movement of the affected hand yet, characteristically persists or even increases during walking.
- with the arms outstretched in front, first with the elbows extended and then flexed with the fingers held in front of the nose. A tremor in this position is called a **postural tremor**. This may be of two types:

  - Physiological tremor: a fine tremor present equally in the two hands. It is enhanced by anxiety, thyrotoxicosis and adrenergic drugs.
  - Essential tremor: this is also usually fine and symmetrical. It persists during movement.

- as the patient repeatedly touches their nose and then your finger with each hand in turn. This manoeuvre elicits an **intention tremor**, a coarse tremor which appears and increases in amplitude as the hand approaches its target. Such a tremor signifies cerebellar dysfunction.

42

Other aspects

What you do next will be determined by what you have found:

- **Resting tremor.** Your aim is to confirm the diagnosis of Parkinson's disease:

  - *Tone.* Test tone in the arms (see introduction). In Parkinson's disease, tone is increased throughout the range of movement. The tremor may also be felt as 'cogwheeling'.
  - *Akinesia.* This is tested by getting the patient to:
    - make piano-playing movements with the index and middle fingers of each hand in turn; or
    - open and close the hand repeatedly with the fingers extended. The amplitude of the movement decreases as the test continues.

      68
    - If these tests are performed only with difficulty, make sure that the problem is not due to weakness. Rapid finger movements are also impaired in patients with hemiparesis but do not show the progressive decrement in amplitude which characterizes this activity in Parkinson's disease. Muscle strength is normal in Parkinson's disease.

  - *Gait.* Check for: loss of arm swing, stooped posture, small steppage and stiffness or hesitation on turning. Eventually, there is loss of balance (demonstrated by performing the 'pull test') and freezing resulting in falls.

    67
  - *Speech.* This will typically be quiet, with a tendency for words to run into each other or to stutter (pallilalia).

    43

- **Postural tremor** (Essential tremor or enhanced Physiological tremor). The aim here is to exclude Parkinson's disease, which is not always easy as in many patients with severe, coarse Essential tremor the tremor persists at rest. Conversely, postural tremor is common in Parkinson's disease. The problem is made more difficult by the fact that patients with Essential tremor may perform piano-playing movements poorly and have cog-wheeling (though on a background of normal tone) when tone is tested. The single most useful way of distinguishing between the two conditions is by *observing the gait*. In Essential tremor the gait is normal; this is never the case in Parkinson's disease (unless they are receiving treatment). In Essential tremor, the face is expressive and the patient gesticulates fluently in conversation. The voice is often tremulous but of good volume. Tremor is often present in unusual sites such as the lips, tongue or chin. Often it is longstanding and there may be a positive family history.

- If it is of recent onset, check for evidence of thyrotoxicosis: tachycardia, sweating, lid lag, exophthalmos, goitre, thyroid bruit, weight loss. Enquire about what drugs the patient is taking.
- **Intention tremor** (cerebellar dysfunction). Look for confirmatory signs of cerebellar dysfunction such as nystagmus, dysarthria and a wide-based unsteady gait. It is important not to confuse this tremor, which *only* appears as the hand approaches its target, with a kinetic tremor ('tremor of movement'). The latter is present in many patients with Essential tremor. The tremor they have in maintaining a posture persists during movement and may even increase as the hand approaches a target; there are no associated cerebellar signs.
- **Less common tremors.** Unfortunately for the candidate, rarities in clinical practice are commonplace in examinations for they often have good signs. It is, therefore, worthwhile to be aware of some of the less common types of tremor:

  - *Dystonic tremor.* Patients with dystonia, such as torticollis, dysphonia or writer's cramp, not uncommonly have an associated tremor. This may have the same distribution as the dystonia (head, voice or hand, respectively, in the examples listed) or involve otherwise unaffected parts of the body. Thus, a patient with torticollis may have a marked tremor of the outstretched hands. Tremors of this type are often coarse, asymmetrical and a little irregular. To complicate matters further, such a 'dystonic tremor' may be present in the head or upper limbs in the absence of any abnormal posturing. Such tremors overlap with Essential tremor.
  - *Holmes (rubral, midbrain or cerebellar outflow) tremor.* This is a coarse, often proximal, tremor of the upper limb which may be present at rest but which increases in amplitude with the arms outstretched and is maximal

when touching a target. The presence of a contralateral oculomotor nerve palsy in some cases points to the midbrain as the likely site of the lesion causing this tremor. It used to be called a 'rubral tremor' on the basis that it arose from the red nucleus of the midbrain, but this is no longer thought to be the case and it has been re-named the Holmes tremor after Gordon Holmes who wrote a definitive description of it.

- **'Bat's wing' tremor.** This refers to a striking, coarse tremor involving the proximal muscles of the upper limb. When this is seen in a young adult you should think of Wilson's disease.[1] Carefully inspect the cornea, illuminated from the side with your torch, for the pathognomonic brown rings (like a brown arcus senilis) described by Kayser[2] and Fleischer[3].

44

45

Box 10.2 TIPS

- If you are wondering whether or not the patient has Parkinson's disease, get them to walk. Patients with Parkinson's disease nearly always fail to swing one or both arms fully. The only exception to this is the occasional patient who is so responsive to levodopa, that, while the drug is working, all signs of the disease disappear.

- If you wish to enhance a resting or postural tremor, in order to observe its characteristics more easily, ask the patient to subtract 7 from 100 and go on subtracting 7s as fast as possible. The stress involved in doing this is guaranteed to increase the tremor.

- Chorea, most types of myoclonus, asterixis and tics differ from tremor in one major way. They are not rhythmical (regular in their timing).

- In Parkinson's disease the amplitude of the tremor is often more marked in one hand than in the other.

- The tremor in Essential tremor, while maximal on holding the arms out, persists during movement and often increases as the finger approaches the target (e.g. the nose).

- A hand tremor which persists during walking is usually due to Parkinson's disease.

Isolated head tremor is never due to Essential tremor. Many such cases have dystonic tremor and a subtle head tilt.

---

1. SA Kinnear Wilson, Queen Square neurologist (1874–1937).
2. Bernard Kayser, German ophthalmologist (1869–1954).
3. Richard Fleischer, German physician (1848–1909).

Other abnormal involuntary movements

11

Inspection
The movement
Differential diagnosis
Drug-induced movement disorders

Likely introduction: 'This patient has noticed some movements of his body. What do you make of them?'

Abnormal involuntary movements can be relatively easy to recognize if you have seen such a case before. In the context of a short case, you may be lucky and recognize it at once. All is not lost if you do not, for more important than jumping to conclusions is your ability to carefully and accurately describe what you see and then come up with a reasonable differential diagnosis.

Inspection

As always, step back and look at the patient as a whole. You have a number of questions in your mind:

- Which parts of the body are involved in the movements (focal, segmental, hemi-, generalized, symmetrical, asymmetrical)?
- What is the patient's posture (head, trunk limbs)?
- What happens to the movements as the patient talks to you? Do they increase or lessen?
- Is the patient relating normally to you?

The movement

In choosing the most appropriate term to describe the movement, it is useful to start off with a general category that does not commit you to a particular diagnosis. Broadly categorize it as *tremor, twitches* or *twisting*:

- **Tremor.** Here, the interval between each movement is relatively constant producing a rhythm with a given frequency and amplitude. Tremor tends to affect a particular part or parts of the body (most commonly the hand). It is the most predictable, easiest to measure, and therefore the easiest to understand of the abnormal involuntary movements. Tremor has been dealt with in the previous chapter and will not be further discussed here. The other movements are less easy to describe and categorize.
- **Twitches** (or **jerks**). Here, the movements are brief, irregular in frequency and amplitude, and often less predictable in their distribution than is the case with tremor. Under this category we may consider the following:
  - *Chorea.* The hallmark of chorea is muscle twitching, usually of low amplitude, which flits in an unpredictable manner from one part of the body to another. It may be briefly rhythmical, causing, for example, the eyebrows to dance. Viewed as a whole, the patient with chorea appears to be in constant motion, restless, as you or I might be waiting for a bus with a full bladder. Yet, they usually do not feel restless and may not even be aware of the movements. Chorea can be generalized or confined to one side of the body (hemi-chorea). Chorea increases when the patient is talking or moving. The gait tends to be lurching and untidy. There is often associated motor impersistence; thus the patient cannot protrude the tongue for more than a few seconds. The causes of chorea are legion and include drugs (neuroleptics and levodopa), Huntington's disease and auto-immune disease such as systemic lupus erythematosus (SLE) and anti-phospholipid syndrome (Box 11.1).

  - *Hemiballismus.* This is a violent jerking, waving, thrusting movement of the proximal arm and leg which usually comes on quite suddenly following a stroke involving the contralateral subthalamic nucleus or its connections. So troublesome are the movements that the patient may sit on the hands to suppress them.

Box 11.1 Management issues in chorea.

Investigations

- Computed tomography (CT)/MRI to exclude infarct/tumour
- Thyroid function tests
- Anti-nuclear factor (ANF), antiphospholipid a/b
- Anti-streptolysin-O-antibody (ASOT)
- Genetic testing for Huntington's disease

Treatment

- Symptomatic
- Tetrabenazine

- *Tics.* Tics most commonly involve the face and head, causing characteristic blinks, grimaces, poutings and head turns; many children have these and grow out of them. When severe, as in some cases of Tourette's[1] syndrome, the whole body may be affected with violent jerks of the shoulders or trunk. The movements tend to lessen with distraction, for example, while talking, but they are voluntarily suppressed only with great difficulty. Tics are best considered as a behavioural disorder. They have a quality which is difficult for the observer to ignore and the movements may spill over into activities which can cause offence or irritation. A cough may be so loud as to make you jump. Sometimes, it is clearly a bark disguised as a cough. Rarely, patients will emit an obscenity or swear word (coprolalia). This is often slipped in mid-sentence (like a tic, which of course it is) rather than delivered with the emphasis that is usually given to swearing. Obscene gestures (copropraxia) are delivered in a similar manner. Patients describe a need or compulsion to make the movement, however embarrassing the context, and experience a sense of relief when it is done. Many of these patients have obsessive compulsive disorder, crippled, for example, by a need to check that the front door is locked even if this requires repeated car journeys.
- *Myoclonus.* This refers to sudden brief 'electric shock-like' muscle twitches which can affect any part of the body. Depending on the setting,

1. *Gilles de la Tourette, French neurologist and pupil of Charcot (1857–1904).*

they may occur spontaneously or also in response to a stimulus such as a noise, touch or pinprick (stimulus-sensitive myoclonus). Myoclonus often increases with voluntary movement. In some cases, the twitches are time-locked to an EEG event and may be regarded as a 'fragment' of an epileptic seizure. The movement is usually associated with a muscular contraction but it can also be caused by gravity as the muscle momentarily loses tone. This is known as **negative myoclonus** or, more commonly, **asterixis** (or in the setting of hepatic failure, **liver flap**).

In hospital practice, myoclonus is seen most commonly in the setting of metabolic disturbance such as diabetic ketoacidosis, post-hypoxic brain injury, epileptic syndromes, and degenerative disease of the brain (e.g. multiple system atrophy) (Box 11.2). The site of origin of myoclonus determines, to some extent, its clinical features:

- *Cortical myoclonus*: low-amplitude, irregular twitches of individual fingers, induced by voluntary movement and sometimes touch or pinprick and associated with giant somatosensory evoked potentials (SSEPs).
- *Brainstem myoclonus*: generalized jerks, affecting the proximal limbs and often triggered by noise.
- *Spinal myoclonus*: semi-rhythmical jerks of the trunk, often involving just a few spinal segments.

Box 11.2 Management issues in myoclonus.

Investigations

- Liver function tests
- Electrolytes and urea
- Glucose
- Electroencephalography (EEG)

Treatment

- Underlying cause
- Drugs: valproate, clonazepam, piracetam

- **Twisting (dystonia).** In dystonia, body parts are twisted into odd *postures* due to abnormal interplay between opposing sets of muscles. In most cases, there are associated *dystonic movements* which may be more or less regular (*dystonic tremor*) or irregular and jerky. A particular subtype of dystonic movement is **athetosis**, which refers to slow, writhing irregular movements of individual fingers and toes and sometimes the face, usually in the setting of cerebral palsy. Dystonia may be *generalized, segmental* (e.g. torticollis and lateral flexion of the trunk), or *focal*. It is usually induced or made worse by voluntary movement, and in some cases only appears with specific activities (e.g. writer's cramp). A key feature in many cases is the presence of a geste antagonistique, whereby, for example, the head posture of a patient with torticollis improves if the patient touches the cheek. (Interestingly, the correction has usually occurred before the hand reaches the face.)

Differential diagnosis

You have reached the point where you have broadly categorized the movement and, hopefully, have some thoughts on the specific type of movement present. Often, the clinical setting in which the movements are occurring makes your task much easier. A middle-aged man with twitches, which you are having difficulty classifying, turns out to have a dementia and strongly positive family history; Huntington's disease now seems likely (Box 11.3). Writhing movements of the limbs which defy classification are readily classified as dopa-induced dyskinesia once you know of the history of Parkinson's disease. Here is a list of conditions to consider:

- **Tremor** (see Chapter 10).
- **Chorea** occurs in a number of settings:

- Huntington's disease

    - Onset usually in early middle age
    - Frontal-type dementia
    - Gaze palsy: blinking to initiate gaze, restricted range of eye movements

---

Box 11.3 Management issues in Huntington's disease.

Investigations

- Computed tomography (CT)/MRI: caudate atrophy
- Thyroid function tests
- Genetic testing (after counselling)

Treatment

- Genetic counselling
- Support for family
- Symptomatic

N.B. Usually do not treat the chorea with tetrabenazine (causes depression and Parkinsonism)

- Akinesia: clumsiness of the hands, untidy gait
- Dystonia: flexed posture
- Positive family history
- Genetic testing

- Auto-immune diseases

  - Systemic lupus erythematosus
    - Commonest cause of chorea in a young woman
    - Often a hemi-chorea
    - Look for typical features:
      - Butterfly rash
      - Arthralgia
      - Renal involvement
    - Blood tests: anti-DNA a/b plus
  - Anti-phospholipid syndrome
    - History of miscarriages
    - History of deep vein thrombosis
    - Blood tests: anti-cardiolipin a/b

- Sydenham's chorea[2]
    - Rare now in First World countries
    - Onset in teens
    - Motor impersistence
    - Fatuous manner may cause erroneous diagnosis of psychogenic disorder
    - Associated rheumatic heart disease
    - Associated with streptococcal throat infection
    - Improves but often persists lifelong in a minor form worsening during pregnancy or with the contraceptive pill

- Blood disorders
    - Polycythaemia rubra vera
        - Often causes hemi-chorea or hemiballismus
    - Neuro-acanthocytosis
        - Rare

- Hyperthyroidism

- **Tics**

- Simple
    - Onset in childhood
    - Single type of tic
    - Often grow out of it

- Tourette's syndrome

    - Onset in childhood
    - Multiple types of tics
    - Persists into adulthood
    - Obsessive Compulsive Disorder

- **Myoclonus**

- Cortical myoclonus

    - Post-hypoxic action myoclonus
    - Spinocerebellar degenerations
    - Coeliac disease

2. *Thomas Sydenham, English physician (1624–1689).*

- Sialidosis (cherry red spot) – rare
- Unverricht[3]-Lundborg (Baltic) myoclonus – rare
- Alzheimer's disease (especially in the setting of Down syndrome)[4]
- Multiple system atrophy (MSA)
- Diffuse Lewy body disease (DLBD)
- Corticobasal degeneration
- Drugs: especially selective serotonin re-uptake inhibitors (SSRIs) (similar appearance, though the site of origin is not known)

- Brainstem myoclonus

  - Metabolic disturbance
  - Diabetic ketoacidosis
  - Renal failure

- Spinal myoclonus

  - Tumour
  - Trauma
  - Radiation

- Some specific myoclonic syndromes

  - Post-hypoxic myoclonus (Lance Adams syndrome)
  - Subacute sclerosing panencephalitis

- **Dystonia.** Many dystonias are now being shown to have a genetic basis. It is conventional, if confusing, to divide dystonias into Primary dystonia, where dystonia is the only abnormality present, and Secondary dystonia, where there are associated neurological features which might include dementia, epilepsy, pyramidal signs, neuropathy, retinopathy, optic atrophy and deafness. The presence of these features helps to narrow the range of diagnostic possibilities.

- Generalized

  - Torsion dystonia
    - Rare
    - Genetic testing DYT1

---

3. *Heinrich Unverricht, German physician (1853–1912).*
4. *James Down, English physician (1828–1896).*

- Segmental (e.g. head and upper limb)

- Focal

  - Cranial
    - Torticollis
      - Anterocollis
        - MSA
        - DLBD
      - Retrocollis
        - Often tardive (drug-induced)
    - Spasmodic dysphonia
    - Blepharospasm
      - Meige[5]
  - Upper limbs

- Task-specific

  - Writer's cramp
  - Musician's cramp

- **Miscellaneous**

- Dystonia/myoclonus

  - Looks like Essential tremor
  - Alcohol-responsive

Drug-induced movement disorders

Having been through the diagnostic process as described, there remains a group of conditions which do not fit readily into the schema above. These are the drug-induced movement disorders. They are more common than most of the conditions considered so far, and in some cases preventable, and for these reasons deserve special consideration.

- **Dopa-induced involuntary movements.** Most patients with Parkinson's disease who respond to levodopa, eventually develop involuntary movements related to the drug regimen. This problem is most marked in younger-onset patients. There are two main types:

5. Henri Meige, French neurologist and student of Charcot (1866–1940).

- *Peak-dose dyskinesia.* About an hour after taking a dose, the patient starts to make writhing twisting movements which are maximal in the trunk and proximal limbs. Often, the patient is unaware or untroubled by the movements. They last for an hour or two, and are made worse by taking another dose of levodopa while they are still present.

- *End-of-dose dystonia.* This occurs as the benefit from a dose of levodopa wears off, or in the early morning before the first dose, and comprises a painful cramping of the toes which makes walking difficult. It is relieved by taking another dose of levodopa.

- **Tardive syndromes.** These were very common before the older-style neuroleptic drugs such as trifluoperazine, chlorpromazine and haloperidol were replaced by the newer neuroleptics such as clozapine, olanzepine and quetiapine. Older patients seem more prone to develop the problem. Inappropriate use of the anti-emetics prochlorperazine, and metoclopramide, as a treatment for dizziness, are a continuing cause of these disabling and preventable disorders. There are several types:

- *Akathisia.* This refers to a feeling of restlessness which is reflected in an inability to sit for any length of time or keep still. The patient paces the floor like a caged tiger. The movements themselves are not abnormal, unlike chorea. It can occur transiently when the older neuroleptics are introduced but may also persist long-term.

- *Tardive dyskinesia.* This mainly affects older patients and is characterized by continuous movements of the mouth, tongue and jaw (bucco-lingual dyskinesia). They are worse when the patient talks. Often they trouble the patient's family more than the patient. Paradoxically, the movements initially get worse when the offending drug is withdrawn and may persist for years thereafter.

- *Tardive dystonia.* This is most commonly seen in young males treated with neuroleptics for schizophrenia. The head is thrown back (retrocollis). Again, the problem is made transiently worse by withdrawal of the drug which caused the problem.

- *Drug-induced parkinsonism.* Neuroleptic drugs may produce a syndrome identical to idiopathic Parkinson's disease. This may persist for a year after the drugs are withdrawn.

Box 11.4 TIPS

- With any involuntary movement, the first decision is whether the movement is rhythmical. If it is not rhythmical, it is better not to call it a tremor.
- The hallmark of chorea is that it is flitting and unpredictable.
- The key to understanding tics is the compulsion that the patient feels before the movement and relief when it is done – Kinnear Wilson likened it to a sneeze.
- The essence of myoclonus is its 'shock-like' quality: a square wave rather than a sinusoid wave. There are exceptions: in subacute sclerosing panencephalitis (SSPE) the jerk is 'hung-up' (sustained).
- Dystonia would be easier to understand if we called it 'dysposture', for it is sustained alteration in posture that sets it apart from the other involuntary movement disorders. Having said that, in some disorders (e.g. torticollis), the postural abnormality is slight and the picture is dominated by dystonic movements.

Speech disturbance

12

Likely introduction: 'Difficulty in speech' or 'Assess this patient's speech'.

In the context of a neurological short case, speech disturbance is likely to be due to *dysarthria* – a problem of articulation, or *aphasia* – a problem of language. The term aphasia is usually reserved for patients with a focal lesion involving the dominant cerebral hemisphere (usually the left, even in left-handed patients) of the brain. Speech may also be impaired in dementia where there is widespread disturbance of function in the cerebral hemispheres (see Chapter 13).

General approach

- Patients with speech disturbance – particularly those with aphasia – find conversation an effort, and easily become distressed. It is important to make the patient feel at ease. Do not stand over them; sit with them. If it is clear that they are struggling, reassure them that you appreciate how upsetting it is not to be able to communicate.
- Engage them in conversation on a topic with which they are likely to feel comfortable: "Tell me about your job (family, holidays, hobbies, etc.)". Your wish is to hear the patient forming sentences, so avoid questions to which the answer is likely to be 'yes' or 'no'. It is often difficult to get a patient to speak freely. In this case, show them a picture (Fig. 12.1) and ask them to describe the scene. This approach has the advantage that you can tell what the patient is trying to say (see below). Do not rush this part of the examination for it forms the basis of your assessment.

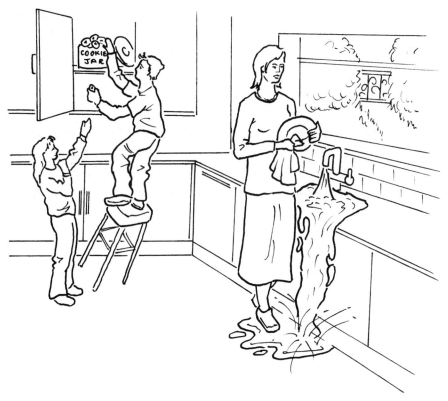

Figure 12.1 A picture which can be shown to an aphasic patient.

- As the patient talks, pay particular attention to three aspects of their speech:
  - are the words normally articulated?
  - is the sentence structure normal?
  - are they using words incorrectly?
- Is there facial asymmetry? Is the right hand used as much as the left? A right hemiparesis often accompanies aphasia.
- Take note of the patient's 'body language'. Patients with non-fluent aphasia often have exaggerated body language. They sigh, gasp, roll their eyes and gesticulate, as they struggle to communicate with you. Sometimes they will burst into tears from sheer frustration. By contrast, patients who cannot communicate because of dementia may be unconcerned or unaware that there is a problem. Their body language is as impoverished as their speech.

You are likely to find one of two main patterns of abnormality, dysarthria or aphasia.

Dysarthria

Here, the words are slurred but the language content – if you were to write it down – is normal. The problem is one of articulation. Slurring of speech signifies weakness or incoordination of the muscles involved in the production of sounds. Common causes are spasticity (e.g. pseudobulbar palsy, motor neurone disease), lower motor neurone bulbar weakness (e.g. progressive bulbar palsy, a form of motor neurone disease) and cerebellar disorders (e.g. multiple sclerosis). Some neurologists can confidently distinguish spastic from cerebellar dysarthria by the quality of speech. I cannot; I therefore rely on the neurological company which the dysarthria keeps.

Faint, quiet (dysphonic) speech is a feature of Parkinson's disease. The voice is also monotonous and the words tend to run into each other. Weakness of the diaphragm and of other respiratory muscles also cause the voice to be quiet.

Assessment of dysarthria involves five steps:

- *Repetition of words or phrases* which are difficult to say. Examples of these include:

  - artillery, constitution, monotonous, constabulary
  - impossibility, autobiography, examination
  - according to legend, statistical analysis.

- Sometimes, a simple word can be correctly articulated but difficulty is encountered as the complexity of the word is progressively increased:

  - Zip, zipper, zippering
  - Please, pleasing, pleasingly
  - City, citizen, citizenship.

- *Repetition of sounds* which test the different muscles of articulation. Where there is weakness of the lips, the patient will have difficulty saying 'puh', of the tongue 'tuh', and of the palate 'kuh'.

- Ask the patient to *cough*. A bovine cough is heard where there is paralysis of a vocal cord due to a recurrent laryngeal nerve palsy.
- Examination of the motor system, in order to determine whether the problem is due to:

  - a lower motor neurone lesion of the muscles of articulation (check for facial weakness; wasting, weakness or fasciculation of the tongue; loss of the gag reflex; palatal palsy).
  - an upper motor neurone lesion of the muscles of articulation (brisk jaw jerk, exaggerated gag reflex, hemiparesis).
  - a cerebellar disturbance (nystagmus, intention tremor of the arms, gait disturbance).
  - an extrapyramidal disorder (check for evidence of Parkinson's disease or other involuntary movement disorders).

- Assessment of whether the patient's problem is more than a failure to articulate words; that they are also aphasic. This is of particular importance in patients presenting with slurred speech and weakness of the right arm, who may have a non-fluent aphasia. In a 'pure' dysarthria, sentence structure, repetition and comprehension will be normal (see below).

Aphasia

This refers to a disturbance in the production or understanding of language, written, spoken and read. It occurs with lesions of the dominant cerebral hemisphere. The main areas of the brain involved in language are shown in Fig. 12.2. As a general rule, lesions of the frontal lobe ('anterior lesions') cause a non-fluent aphasia with preservation of comprehension. This is traditionally known as an 'expressive' or 'motor' aphasia. Lesions of the parietal and temporal lobes ('posterior lesions') cause a fluent aphasia and there is impairment of comprehension. The traditional term for this is 'receptive' or 'sensory' aphasia. Assessment of aphasia involves three steps.

1. Is the speech fluent, or non-fluent?

In a **non-fluent aphasia**, the patient's speech is effortful and may be slurred. Sentences are short and lack 'filler' words such as 'and', 'the', 'so' and 'to'. The

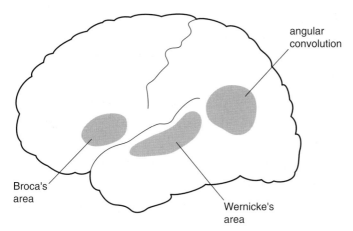

Figure 12.2 The main language areas.

information content is often high. If you write down what is said, the result looks like a telegram – for example, "Come hospital get better". The normal melody (prosody) of speech is lost, and the patient often appears to be making an exaggerated effort to get the words out.

In a **fluent aphasia**, words flow freely, sentences are of a normal length, the voice rises and falls melodiously, but the information content is low. What is said is difficult to understand and words are used wrongly. When shown Fig. 12.1, such a patient might say, "The little boys and girls are getting up a stool and putting some cookies, right? Ah, this is the trouble the sing, the sing is overflowing, right?" Wrong words are known as paraphasias and are of three types:

- phonemic paraphasia: a consonant is substituted causing, for example, the patient to say 'sing' when they mean 'sink'.
- semantic paraphasia: a word is changed for another with an obvious association, e.g. a knife is called a fork.
- neologism: a non-existent word is substituted for the intended word, e.g. a 'room' is called a 'boof'. Paraphasic errors usually signify involvement of the posterior speech areas. In mild cases, speech may be normal for a few sentences and then the sentence structure breaks down and paraphasias appear.

2. Is the patient able to repeat?

Patients with aphasia often have difficulty repeating the phrase 'no ifs, ands or buts'. They will say 'no ands or buts' or 'no ifs and buts', but never the full phrase. Words which are readily linked to a visual image, such as house, ship, book, face and cigarettes, can often be repeated without difficulty. It is thought that the memory stores of these words have a wider distribution within the brain than non-picture words, and are therefore less likely to be affected by lesions confined to the speech area. The inability to repeat is used in some classifications of aphasia which attempt to relate the type of aphasia with the site of the lesion. In practice, the main value of testing repetition is in confirming that the patient is aphasic.

3. Does the patient have normal comprehension?

Patients with severe disturbance of comprehension often give the appearance that they fully understand everything that is said to them and, indeed, may think that they do understand. They smile or nod when there is a pause in the conversation. They gesticulate so convincingly that their problem may initially go unnoticed by their own family. These patients have normal body language, taking their cues from the movements of those around them and responding appropriately. In testing their comprehension, one must make allowance for the fact that they may not be able to find the words to tell you that they understand what is being said to them. This is done in two ways:

- reduce the amount of language that they need to use to the minimum: 'yes' or 'no'. Ask a sequence of questions: 'Are you in hospital?'; 'Are we sitting in your house?'; 'Have you got pyjamas on?'; 'Have you got a coat on?' Remember that the patient has an even chance, each time, of giving the correct response. Ask a number of questions, therefore, and vary them so that there are no sequences in which the same answer, 'Yes' or 'No', would be correct. Perseveration is common in aphasia, causing the patient to repeat the same response several times. Subtle defects of comprehension may only be picked up by asking 'double-barrelled' questions: 'Do you put your shoes on before your socks?'; 'Do you put your socks on before your shoes?'; 'Do you shut the car door before getting into the car?'; 'If the lion ate the tiger, is the tiger alive?'

Table 12.1 Current definitions of aphasia.

Speech type*	Repetition	Comprehension	Associated signs
Non-fluent			
Broca's[1] aphasia	Impaired/normal	Normal	Weakness R arm
Global aphasia	Impaired	Impaired	R hemiparesis
Fluent			
Wernicke's aphasia	Impaired	Impaired	Homonymous hemianopia
Conduction aphasia	Impaired	Normal	
Isolation aphasia	Normal	Impaired	
Nominal aphasia	Normal	Normal	

*After Geschwind MD. Aphasia. *N Engl J Med* 1971; 654–656.

- Ask the patient to obey commands: 'Touch your nose' or 'Touch your knee'. Many patients with aphasia can obey single commands, but cannot follow sequences: 'Touch your chin, then your nose, then your ear'. Patients with normal comprehension are often unable to protrude the tongue on command due to an apraxia.

To summarize, in describing an aphasia you should state whether it was fluent or non-fluent, whether there were paraphasic errors, and whether repetition and comprehension were impaired. A description such as this is probably more useful than terms such as 'nominal aphasia' or 'Wernicke's aphasia', which mean different things to different people. If you wish to use these terms, Table 12.1 provides a guide to their current usage.

To complete the examination, one should ask the patient to read and to write. The information obtained from doing this is similar to that gained from listening to the speech. Patients with non-fluent aphasias have great difficulty writing at all – even with the left hand. Patients with fluent aphasia make paraphasic errors in their reading and writing.

1. *Pierre-Paul Broca, French anatomist and surgeon (1824–1880).*

Box 12.1 TIPS

- In a short case, you are doing well if you can say, with good evidence, that the patient is aphasic. The subdivisions of aphasia, outlined in Table 12.1, are less important, for many patients do not fit comfortably into this or any other system of classification. Thus, it is not uncommon for patients – for example with a posterior lesion – to have marked poverty of speech, albeit well articulated.

- The left hemisphere is dominant for language in the majority of individuals, regardless of their handedness.

- A fluent aphasia, with normal comprehension and repetition (nominal aphasia), is characteristically seen in metabolic encephalopathies.

- Gerstmann's[2] syndrome (finger agnosia, agraphia, acalculia and right–left disorientation) is a favourite diagnosis of many candidates faced with a patient with aphasia. There is, of course, little point in testing for these features in a patient who has severely impaired comprehension.

- In children, aphasia is always non-fluent, regardless of the site of the lesion.

- How do you assess the quality of speech in a severely aphasic patient who is almost mute? Get the patient to count to 10, calling out the first few numbers with him and 'conducting' them through the remainder by hand signals.

- It is common for candidates to miss impairment of comprehension through inadequate testing. They will hurriedly ask the patient to point out different body parts (hand, foot, elbow) while looking at the part in question. This may give the patient who is relying solely on body language all the help they need to perform the task.

---

2. Josef Gerstmann, Austrian neuropsychiatrist (1887–1969).

Higher function testing

13

General approach
Formal cognitive testing
Some syndromes of dementia

Likely introduction: 'Perform higher function testing in this patient' or 'Assess this patient for the presence of dementia or cognitive impairment'.

It is most unlikely – and probably unfair – for you to be expected to perform a short case assessment in a patient with dementia who might well have difficulty conforming to the constraints of such an exercise in the limited time available. Testing higher function is, nevertheless, a most important part of the neurological examination, and it as well to have a scheme which you follow where the issue of cognitive impairment arises. You could be asked to perform this on a cooperative subject in the neurology short case. What follows is an account of how you would approach a patient with cognitive impairment in Casualty.

General approach

As with the aphasic patient, your approach to the patient with cognitive impairment will make allowance for the fact that there are problems of communication and the patient is anxious or alarmed. Sit beside the patient and make every effort by your manner to put them at their ease. If the answers they give are to questions you didn't ask, be patient and resist the temptation to be hectoring in your efforts to gain more information. Better still, have a relative or friend present who can provide moral support and fill in the aspects of the history which the patient is unable to provide; patients with dementia often lack insight into their problem.

- **Delirium versus dementia.** One of your first tasks is to determine whether this is an acute potentially reversible problem of *delirium* or a longer-term problem of *dementia*. Of course, the patient may have both: patients with dementia are more prone to delirium if they develop, for example, an infection. As you begin to examine the patient, make note of certain key findings:

  - *Grooming*: if the patient is unkempt with long unwashed hair and decayed teeth, the problem is likely to be long-standing, in keeping with a history of dementia.
  - *Bruising*: note any facial bruising or black eyes, feel over the scalp for boggy swelling (over a skull fracture), and look behind the ears for the tell-tale bruising of Battle sign (base of skull fracture). Any evidence of head trauma will encourage you to perform the CT scan of the head earlier rather than later; you do not want delay diagnosing a subdural haematoma.
  - *Level of consciousness*: dementia itself is not a cause of drowsiness. If the patient keeps falling asleep or is hard to rouse, you are dealing with delirium, most commonly due to *drug or alcohol overdose*, *infection* or *metabolic disturbance*. Delirious patients may go through periods of arousal in which they shout, moan or become aggressive. At these times, they may pluck restlessly at the sheets.
  - *Pulse, blood pressure, respiration*. Sweating, tachycardia, swings in blood pressure and altered breathing patterns are all common in delirium.

- **Behaviour:** patients with frontal dementia, once it has passed the early stages, often display *aspontaneity*. They have no complaints and do not initiate conversation. They sit or lie quite happily doing nothing, and showing no frustration. They are orientated, particularly for surroundings, and their responses to your questions may be sensible and appropriate, leading you to the erroneous conclusion that there is not much wrong with them. Such patients often show *environmental dependence*: they are unable to inhibit their innate or acquired responses to external stimuli. Exploratory behaviour with the hands and mouth (grasping and groping), visual fixation and following, using objects (utilization behaviour) and mimicry are behaviours which are controlled by the frontal lobes. When the frontal lobes are not functioning normally, such behaviours are exhibited indiscriminately. They can be readily tested:

- *Grasping and groping.* Hold your index and middle fingers in a vertical plane (i.e. NOT in a normal 'hand-shaking' posture) close to the patient's hand. When they see the hand, they will reach out and grasp it.

  The grasp reflex is tested by sliding your index and middle fingers across the palm of the hand. This is sometimes distinguished from the traction reflex where you run your fingers along the length of the patient's fingers – from base to tip – again causing him or her to grasp them. The latter is said to induce the response by inducing a stretch reflex in the finger flexors and will be positive in a patient with hyper-reflexia of the upper limbs and no frontal lobe dysfunction. In practice, they provide very similar information. If the patient grips your fingers, ask him not to. Often, this will inhibit the response, but when you repeat the manoeuvre a few moments later, or after distraction, the grasping returns. A similar response is seen if you approach the patient's mouth with your index finger (after apologizing for the intrusion); the mouth opens and the patient may move the head forward to grasp the finger.

  Such patients may also have forced visual following; in contrast to their general lack of activity, their eyes follow you as you move around the room or bed. If you move your penlight in a circle in front of them, they will follow it, even when asked not to.

- *Utilization behaviour.* Offer the patient your own or a colleague's glasses. The normal response is one of surprise. Patients with frontal lobe disinhibition will put them on, and a second and even a third pair if they are offered. If you give them your stethoscope they may attempt to use it. These patients tend to fiddle endlessly with whatever catches their attention: dressing gown cord, bed head, sheets.

- *Imitation behaviour (mimicry).* While conversing, put your arm out or up and hold it for a few seconds. The patient with frontal disinhibition will tend to copy you. This, incidentally, is not an aspect of the examination you will want to try on patients with normal cognition!

Formal cognitive testing

The Mini-Mental State is now used routinely in most hospitals. With its emphasis on orientation and memory (it was designed as a screening test for

Alzheimer's disease[1]), it is not a sensitive test of frontal lobe function. Evidence of frontal lobe dysfunction is best gained from the history given by the family: loss of insight, inappropriate behaviour, impairment of judgement in financial and personal matters, and loss of the ability to organize home or work activities. These are difficult things for the non-expert to gauge, particularly when there are severe time constraints. The features of aspontaneity and release of behaviours outlined above only become apparent in moderately advanced cases of frontal dementia. What follows is an abbreviated and modified version of the Addenbrooke's Cognitive Examination (Fig. 13.1). In the short case examination, this will provide you with a flavour of the sort of problems the patient may be experiencing in: orientation, memory, verbal fluency, language and visuospatial sense.

Some syndromes of dementia

By definition, in dementia, there is impairment of memory and deficits in at least one other cognitive domain (speech, praxis, executive function, or visuospatial function) sufficient to produce occupational or social disability. The pattern of abnormality varies according to which part of the brain is affected:

- **Alzheimer's syndrome** (Box 13.1)

  - Initially, impairment of memory
  - Later extends to all other domains: spatial sense, language, frontal executive function

- **Dementia of frontal lobe type**

  - Initially, change in behaviour with loss of social skills, loss of verbal fluency
  - Later, loss of organizational skills, judgement
  - Eventually, aspontaneity and frontal release behaviour
  - Three sub-types of frontal dementia are recognized:

    - Dorsolateral: executive dysfunction
    - Orbitofrontal: disinhibition
    - Medial: akinetic mutism

---

1. *Alois Alzheimer, German pathologist (1864–1915).*

Selected Tests modified from the Addenbrooke's Cognitive examination	Patient's name DOB MRN Date	
ORIENTATION Year? .... Month? .... Day of the week?	Country? .... State/County? .... Hospital? .... Floor?	
ANTEROGRADE MEMORY Repeat this name and address and flower Peter Marshall 42 Market St Newcastle Daffodil (Test recall after 5 minutes)	RETROGRADE MEMORY Name of PM? USA President?	
	ATTENTION Say the months backwards	
LANGUAGE Ask the patient to: give the name for the hands of your watch, the sole of your shoe, the nib of your pen	Point to the door, floor and ceiling	Repeat 'No ifs, ands, or buts'
APRAXIA Ask the patient to mime holding a piece of paper with the left hand and to cut it with a pair of scissors in the right hand. If he/she makes scissoring movements with the index and middle fingers, remind him that he/she is holding the scissors. If he/she has difficulty, repeat with real paper and scissors		
VERBAL FLUENCY Tell me as many words as you can think of beginning with the letter P, but not people or places. You have one minute to go. (>9)	Tell me the names of as many animals as you can think of in 1 minute, beginning with any letter of the alphabet. (>17)	
VISUOSPATIAL ABILITIES Ask the patient to copy your drawing of a cube	Draw a circle and ask the patient to fill in the numbers of the clock	

Figure 13.1 Modified version of the Addenbrooke's Cognitive Examination.

Box 13.1 Management issues in dementia.

Investigations

- Computed tomography (CT)/MRI to exclude infarct/tumour
- Cerebral single-photon emission computed tomography (SPECT) scan
- Thyroid function tests
- Vitamin B$_{12}$, folate
- Infections: syphilis, HIV
- Liver function tests (LFTs) and electroencephalography (EEG) to exclude hepatic encephalopathy
- Venereal Disease Research Laboratories (VDRL) tests, HIV

Treatment

- Symptomatic
- Carer support, home modifications
- Respite care
- Antidepressants
- Anti-cholinesterase drugs

- **Dementia in Parkinsonism**

- Occurs only after many years in idiopathic Parkinson's disease when it causes slowing of thinking, loss of verbal fluency, visual hallucinations and paranoid delusions (often at night) with good preservation of social skills. One of the clues that the patient is developing cognitive impairment is the appearance of apraxia of the hands. They cannot accurately copy the movement you demonstrate to test akinesia.

  They cannot copy you when you make a cut, fist and slap motion with one hand on the other (Luria test).[2]

  They cannot mime slicing a loaf of bread with a knife or cutting a piece of paper with a pair of scissors without using the hand as the tool (even when corrected) or making errors in the sequence of movements or position that the limbs adopt.

2. Aleksander Romanovich Luria, Russian aphasiologist (1902–1977).

- Diffuse Lewy Body Disease: here, similar features occur early in the course of the Parkinsonism:
- Dementia of frontal lobe type is prominent from the onset of progressive supranuclear palsy (PSP).

- **Vascular dementia**

  - Hypertension
  - Stepwise progression
  - Emotional lability
  - Pseudobulbar palsy with brisk jaw jerk
  - Marche à petit pas

- **Treatable/preventable causes of dementia**

  - Hypothyroidism: may be drowsy, puffy face, slow relaxing reflexes
  - Depression ('pseudo-dementia')
  - Vitamin B_{12} deficiency: absent ankle jerks
  - Wernicke-Korsakoff dementia[3]

    - Eye signs may improve with thiamine, the dementia does not
    - Confabulation is a feature

  - AIDS
  - Syphilis
  - Systemic lupus erythematosus (SLE)
  - Frontal meningioma

Box 13.2 TIPS

- If a confused patient is drowsy, the immediate problem is likely to be one of delirium, not dementia.
- The most useful aspect of the clinical assessment is the history obtained from the patient's relatives or spouse.
- The Mini-Mental State Examination does not adequately test frontal lobe function.
- The earliest feature of frontal lobe dysfunction which is readily tested is impairment of verbal fluency (generation of words).

---

3. Sergei Sergeyovich Korsakoff, Russian neuropsychiatrist (1854–1900).

- Signs of advanced frontal lobe dysfunction include aspontaneity, grasping and groping, utilization behaviour and forced mimicry.
- The patient who is worried that he/she might have Alzheimer's disease rarely does: loss of insight is an early feature of dementia in Alzheimer's disease.
- Always run through the check list of reversible dementias.
  - 'Pseudo-dementia' due to depression.
  - Hypothyroidism.
  - Vitamin B_{12} deficiency.
  - Frontal meningioma.
- When discussing memory, the old classification of short- and long-term memory loss is no longer adequate. Show that you are familiar with the following terms:

- *Declarative memory*: all the facts that you are able to recall, comprising:

  - *Episodic (autobiographical) memory*: events in your own life linked to a specific time and place.
  - *Semantic memory*: the body of general knowledge, linguistic skills and vocabulary which you have acquired.

- *Procedural memory*: the memory of motor skills you have acquired.
- *Working memory*: the ability to retain the information necessary to complete a task or to hold a conversation.

CD Videos Index

Video 11. Antalgic gait and positive Trendelenburg sign in a patient with left sacro-ileitis. She minimizes the time that she bears weight on the painful left leg while walking by hurrying through with the stride on the right. When weight-bearing in the standing position, the pelvis momentarily sags on the right due to failure of the left hip abductors to hold the weight.

Video 12. Gait in advanced Parkinson's disease. Difficulty getting out of the chair; flexed at the hips; walks slowly with no arm swing; paradoxically, she can still run.

Video 13. Pull test with retropulsion in Parkinson's disease. The patient walks well, though with absent arms swing. Runs backwards when pulled from behind.

Video 14. Marche à petit pas due to multiple lacunes (seen on MRI). Small steps, festination (hurrying) when turning and negotiating the doorway. Like parkinsonism, but with a broadened base.

Video 15. Marche à petit pas due to normal-pressure hydrocephalus. Pre-shunt. The patient walks with small steps on a wide base with preserved arm swing and upright posture.

Video 16. The same patient as in Video 14, walking normally after being shunted.

Video 17. Mild cerebellar ataxia. Broad-based, unsteady on turning, uneven stride.

Video 18. Gait in cervical dystonia. The head is tilted to the right as the patient walks.

Video 19. Gait in Torsion dystonia. The patient walks awkwardly and hurriedly with the right arm internally rotated, the left arm flexed at the elbow, the right foot dorsiflexed, and the head tilted to the right.

Video 20. Gait in Huntington's disease. The patient has a curious, untidy, mannered way of walking: bending the knees, pausing, and making choreiform movements with his fingers.

Video 21. Gait in dopa-induced dyskinesia. As the patient walks, he makes continuous writhing twisting movements of his head, trunk and limbs.

Video 22. Long-standing right facial palsy. Deepened right naso-labial fold; spontaneous blinking stronger on the normal (left) side; right corner of the mouth twitches when he blinks; smiling, pouting or blowing his cheeks out all cause the right eye to close; right cheek blows out less than left (tighter right buccinator). All features of overactivity of surviving axons in the right facial nerve associated with synkinesis ('cross-talk' between axons). These signs are not due to contracture of the right facial muscles as they are lost if the nerve is severed by, for example, surgery for acoustic neuroma.

Video 23. Right upper motor neurone facial palsy following stroke. The patient's face is symmetrical at rest; on being asked to smile, he blinks and closes his eyes (apraxia of smiling) and then fails to elevate the right angle of the mouth fully; later, when amused, he smiles symmetrically.

Video 24. Bell's palsy. The patient is unable to raise the right eye brow (frontalis), or screw up the right eye (orbicularis oculi), or smile on the right, or purse his lips on the right (orbicularis oris) or contract the right platysma. When he screws the eyes up, the right eye is seen to roll up (Bell's sign).

Video 25. Facial and gaze palsy due to pontine metastasis. Widened left palpebral fissure; not blinking on left; loss of left naso-labial fold; unable to raise left eyebrow (frontalis); unable to screw up left eye (orbicularis oculi); left cheek blows out (buccinator weakness); able to look to the right but not the left (left gaze palsy). CT: multiple lesions including one in the left pons.

Video 26. Selective right facial weakness from skin cancer. The right upper lip fails to purse, and the patient is unable to form a seal with his mouth when attempting to blow out his cheeks; he is able to raise his eyebrows and screw up his eyes normally; unable to flare the right nostril. The scar on the right cheek is from previous surgery for squamous cell carcinoma.

Video 27. Left oculomotor (IIIrd) nerve palsy with pupillary sparing. Complete ptosis; the patient is unable to fully adduct left eye on right lateral gaze; then fixates with left eye, causing right eye to abduct (Hering's law); normal abduction with left eye but limited elevation. Pupils equal.

Video 28. Unilateral ptosis due to myasthenia gravis. Ptosis increases with sustained upward gaze and improves after a brief rest.

Video 29. Marked left ptosis, bilateral ophthalmoplegia and weakness of orbicularis oculi in Kearns–Sayre syndrome.

Video 30. Ocular myasthenia gravis. Ptosis and divergent squint; on sustained upward gaze, the ptosis increases; later the ptosis is abolished by injection of edrophonium.

Video 31. Early Progressive Supranuclear Gaze Palsy (Steele Richardson syndrome). The patient's range of voluntary eye movements is good, but his vertical saccades, particularly when looking down, are slow.

Video 32. Left abducens (VI) nerve palsy. The left eye fails to abduct on left lateral gaze.

Video 33. Right trochlear (IV) nerve palsy. The head is tilted to the left; on left lateral gaze, the right eye rides up – this is more marked when the head is tilted to the right and corrected by tilting the head to the left.

Video 34. Left internuclear ophthalmoplegia. On right lateral gaze, the left eye fails to fully adduct and the right eye overshoots and then makes correcting nystagmoid movements.

Video 35. Parinaud's syndrome. On attempted upward gaze the eyes jerk rhythmically towards each other.

Video 36. Parinaud's syndrome. On attempted upward gaze, the eyes retract rhythmically into the orbits.

Video 37. Horizontal nystagmus. On left lateral gaze there is horizontal nystagmus with the fast phase to the left; on right lateral gaze there is horizontal nystagmus with the fast phase to the right.

Video 38. Vertical nystagmus on downward gaze, fast phase down.

Video 39. Horizontal pendular nystagmus. This is present continuously in the primary position and increases in amplitude on lateral gaze. No fast and slow phase.

Video 40. Resting tremor in Parkinson's disease. Coarse resting pill-rolling tremor in hands. Chin tremor.

Video 41. Postural tremor in Essential tremor. Fine tremor of the outstretched arms; this goes when the arms are at rest and persists during movement; no akinesia of the hands.

Video 42. Intention tremor in cerebellar disease. The patient develops a coarse tremor of the hand as her finger approaches her nose, especially on the right side; there is clumsiness (ataxia) of the hands when she slaps her thighs.

Video 43. Speech in Parkinson's disease. A quiet voice with a tendency to stutter (pallilalia).

Video 44. Holmes tremor. Coarse postural and intention tremor in a patient with midbrain lesion.

Video 45. Bat's wing tremor in a patient with Wilson's disease. At rest, he has a head tremor (titubation); with the arms abducted at the shoulder and flexed at the elbow, he develops a coarse asymmetrical proximal tremor of the arms.

Video 46. Non-fluent aphasia following intracerebral haemorrhage from a left hemisphere arteriovenous malformation (AVM). The patient exerts great effort to get any words out, and there are long pauses during which he gesticulates and appears to be frustrated; his sentences are short and easy to understand; his comprehension is normal.

Video 47. Fluent aphasia in a man with a left parietal glioma. He speaks freely with well-formed sentences and normal prosody (melody), at times making no mistakes; he then gets stuck '. . . and then for an extent for a week I was a problem with poising . . . voicing'. He appears to understand what is said to him but has great difficulty identifying and touching parts of his face in sequence. He is unable to repeat. In summary, he has a fluent aphasia with impaired comprehension and repetition and he makes paraphasic errors.

Video 48. Wernicke's aphasia following a cardioembolic stroke. The patient speaks freely, but what he says is so littered with paraphasias as to make it almost impossible to understand. His comprehension is poor.

Video 49. Chorea in Huntington's disease. This patient makes constant twitching movements of her hands and feet; she grimaces and her eyebrows dance. All this increases when she talks.

Video 50. Hemiballismus. There are almost continuous irregular coarse jerks of the proximal part of the left arm which persist/increase during hand movement and walking.

Video 51. Tourette's syndrome. Blinking, grimacing, and platysma contraction are seen, particularly when the patient talks.

Video 52. Post-hypoxic myoclonus. At rest, this patient is still, but when she raises her arms or legs, large-amplitude, shock-like jerks are seen. The jerks interfere with her attempt to touch a pointer, but there is no true intention tremor.

Video 53. Asterixis. The outstretched hands and fingers repeatedly drop and then recover, reflecting a momentary loss of tone.

Video 54. Mini-myoclonus. There are fine, shock-like lateral movements of individual fingers.

Video 55. Generalized dystonia. The patient's head is turned to the right and the mouth pulls to the left as he talks. The fingers of the left hand are splayed, and the left elbow and wrist are flexed. All actions are interrupted by slow involuntary movements of his limbs and neck.

the tremor is pill-rolling, the thumb rubbing against the index. A side-to-side tremor of similar frequency is seen in the jaw.

Video 66. Intention tremor. A coarse (high-amplitude, low-frequency) tremor is seen in the right hand as the index finger approaches the pointer and the patient's nose.

Video 67. Falls in Parkinson disease. The patient walks cautiously with small steps and with a coarse tremor of the right hand. When he crosses the shadow thrown by light coming through the doorway, he freezes and falls to his knees.

Video 68. Tremor, akinesia and gait in Parkinson's disease. While sitting, there is a coarse tremor of the right hand, causing flexion and extension at the wrist. The tremor pauses briefly when he raises the arms. There is slowing of voluntary flexion and extension of the hands (bradykinesia). The chin shakes. He does not swing the (tremulous) right arm on walking.

Video 69. Groping. The patient reaches out and grasps the hands which are offered to him (even though he has been asked not to) and is unable to let go. He also grasps with his feet.

Video 70. Mouth grasp. This patient flexes her head and opens her mouth to an approaching finger even when asked not to.

Video 71. Forced visual following (visual grasping). The patient follows the light with her eyes, even though it circles uncomfortably. She is unable to suppress the behaviour.

Video 72. Utilization behaviour. The patient stacks three pairs of spectacles on his nose, one at a time, as each is offered to him.

Video 73. Forced mimicry. When the examiner raises his hand with two fingers extended, the patient incorporates the posture into his own gestures. He also imitates left arm raising, both arm raising, right fist clenching and left leg raising, while continuing the conversation.

Video 74. Apraxia in Parkinson's disease. This patient is unable to copy accurately the akinesia test for Parkinsonism, flexing the interphalangeal joints as well as the metacarpophalangeal joints.

Video 75. Luria test. The patient is not able to follow the sequence of fist, cut and slap.

Video 76. Miming in apraxia. The patient is able to obey a simple sequence of pointing commands (showing that her comprehension is reasonable), but is unable to mime cutting a loaf.

Video 77. Dressing apraxia. The patient gets into a tangle trying to put her jacket back on, having inadvertently pulled the left sleeve inside out.

Index